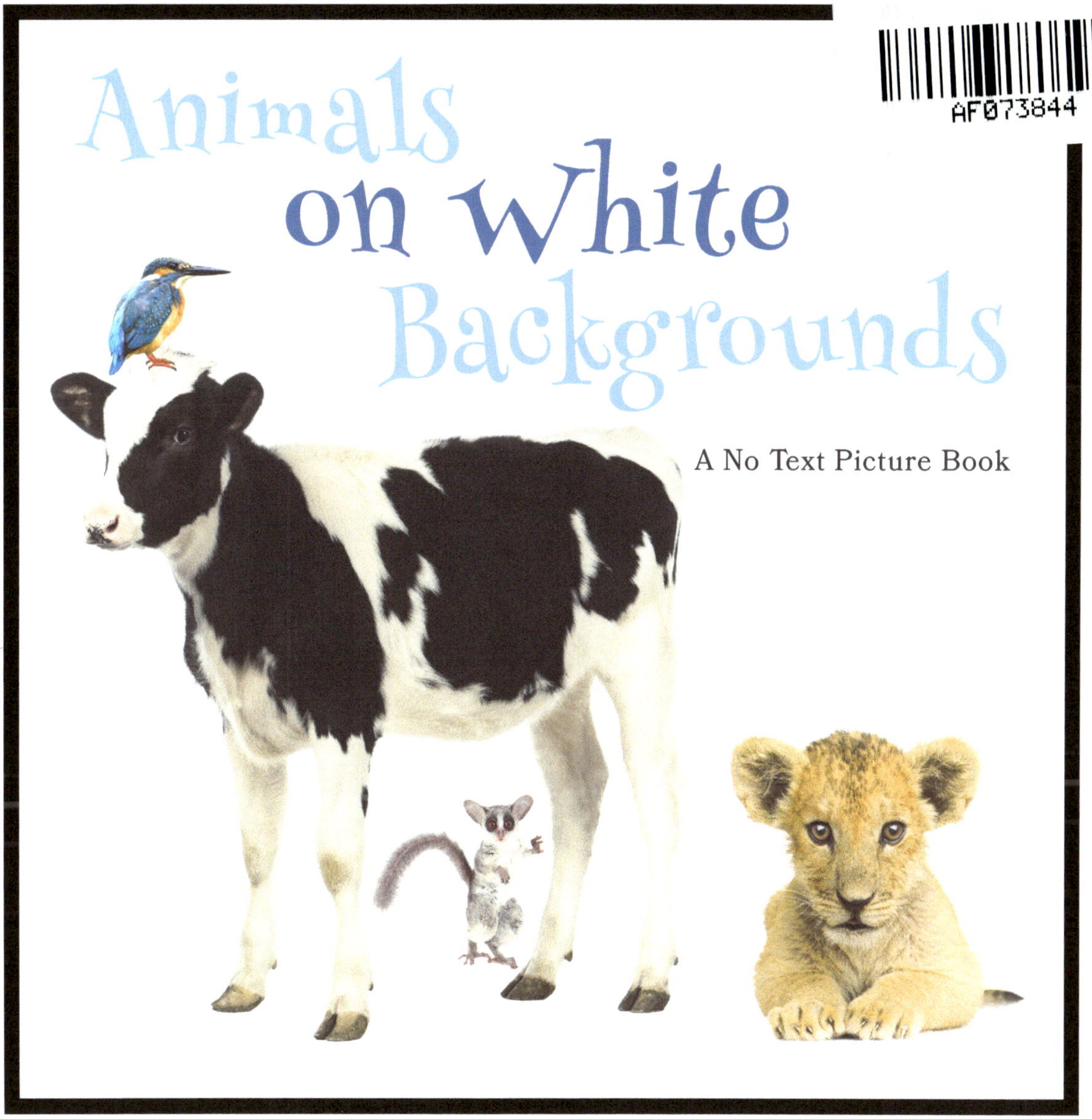

Animals on White Backgrounds

A No Text Picture Book

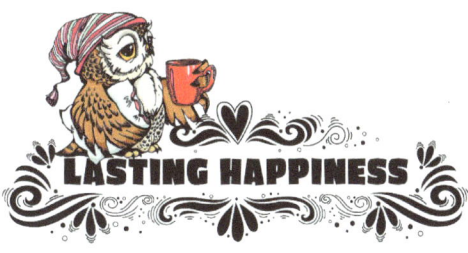

© 2021 Lasting Happiness | All rights reserved.
No part of this book may be reproduced or copied in any manner without prior written permission from the publisher.

ISBN: 9798746805737

To:

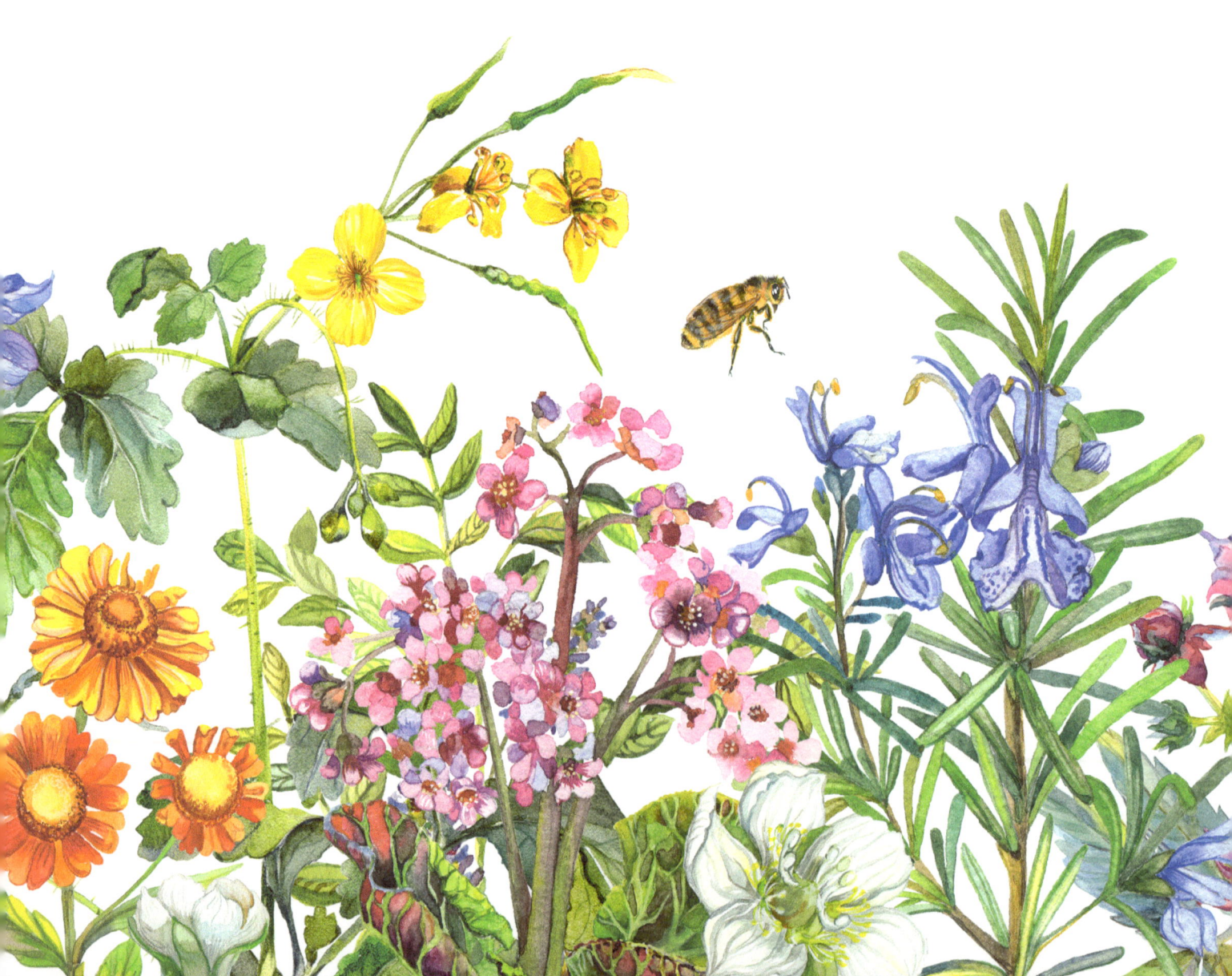

From:

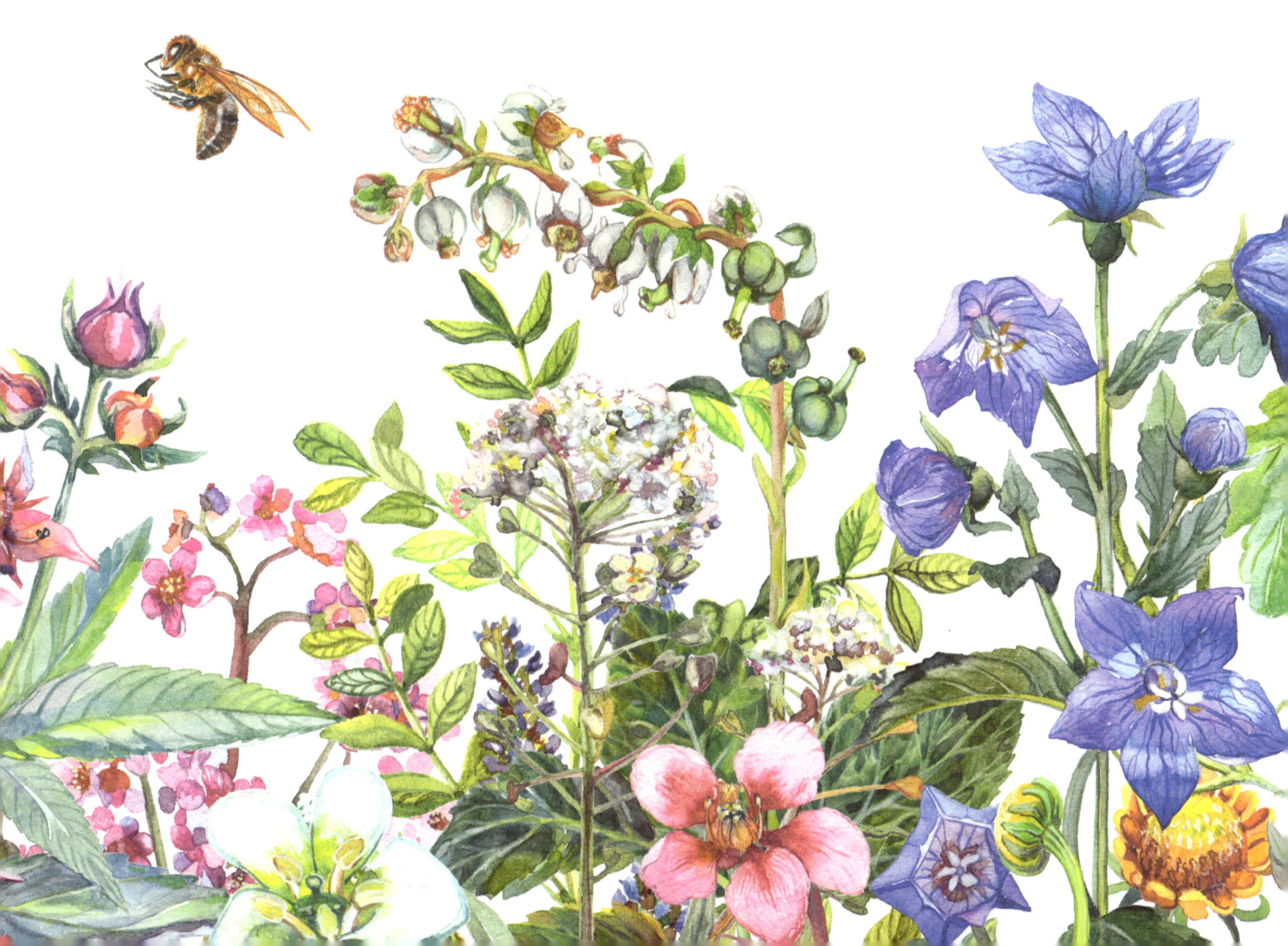

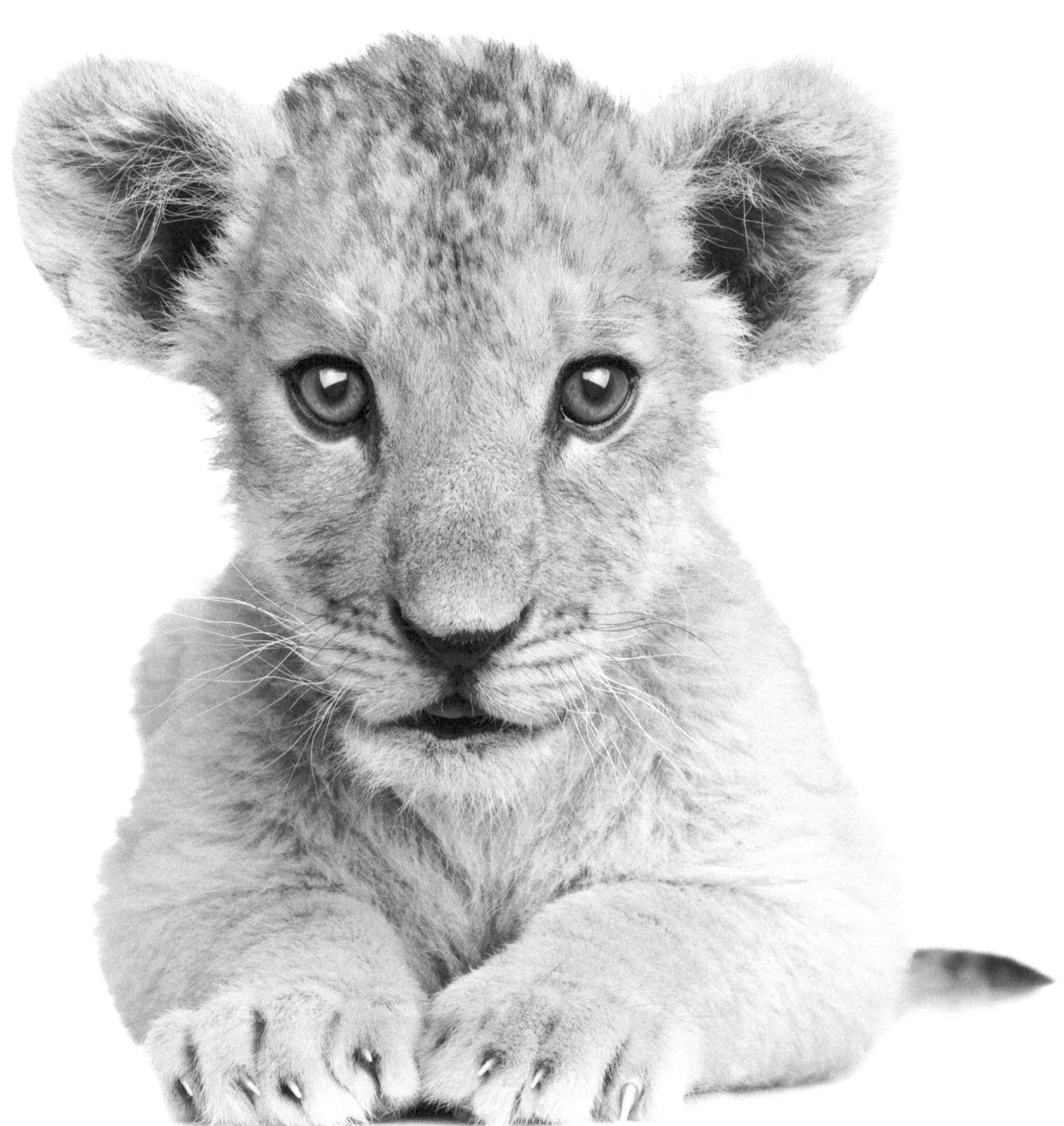

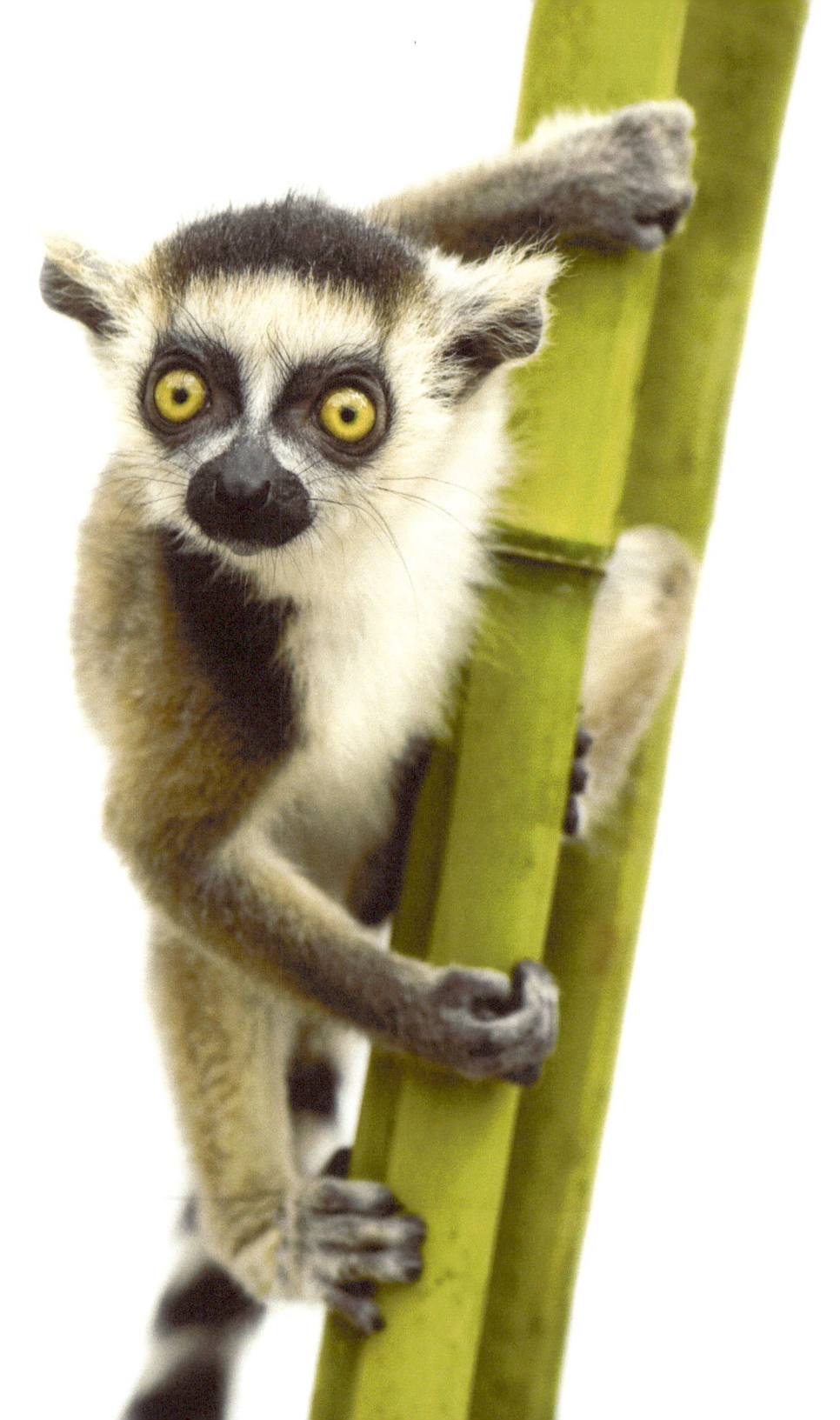

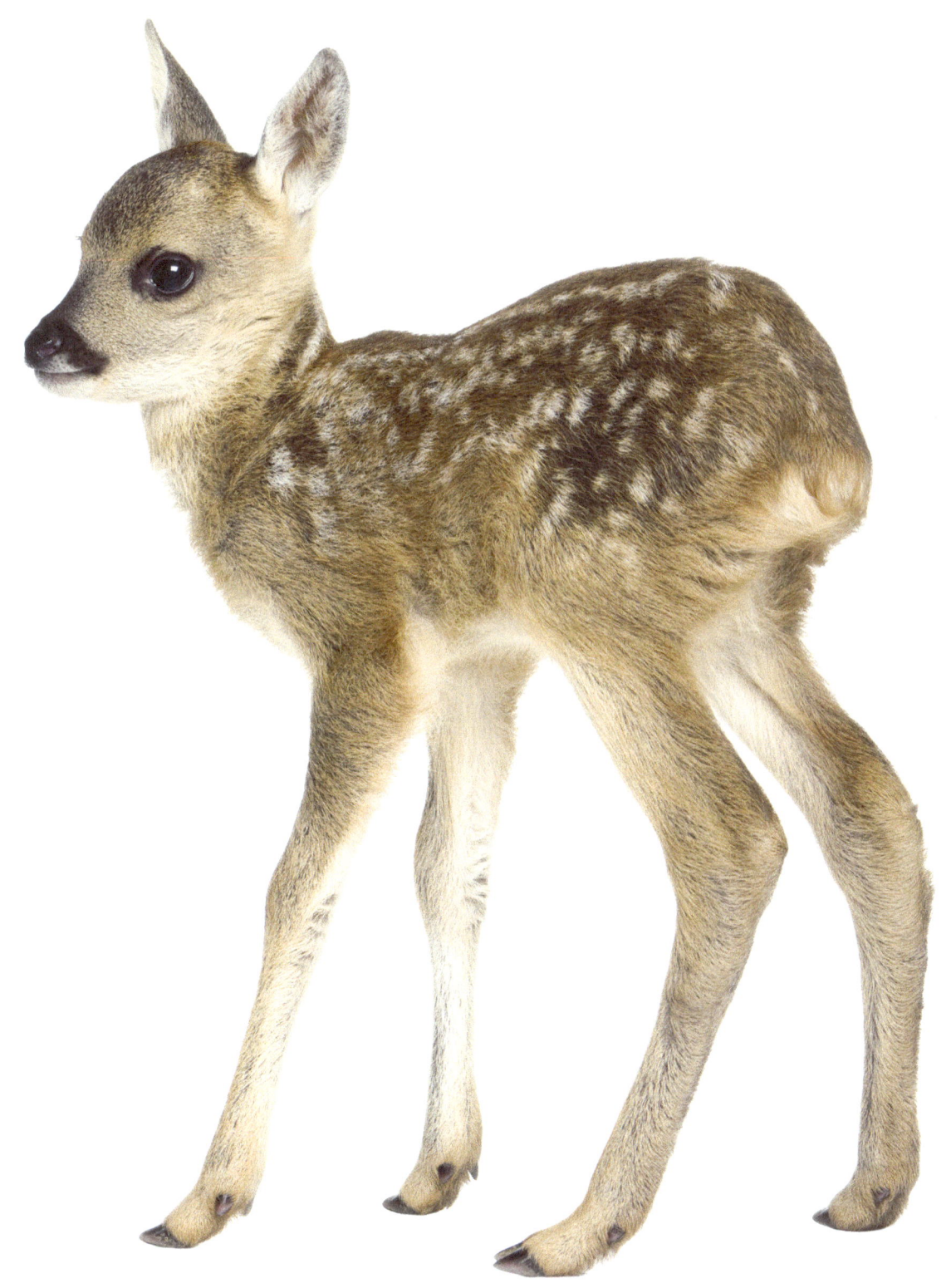

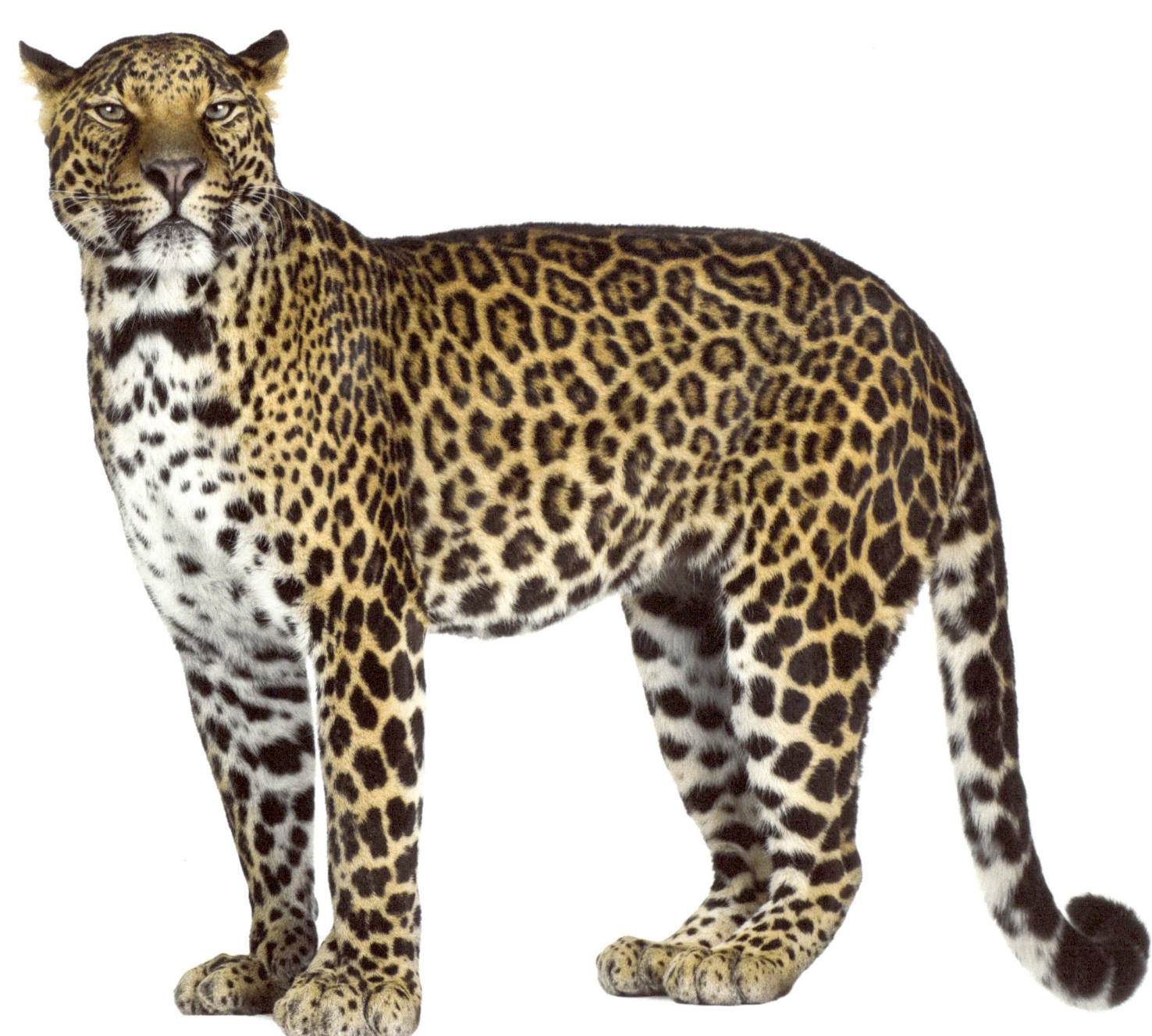

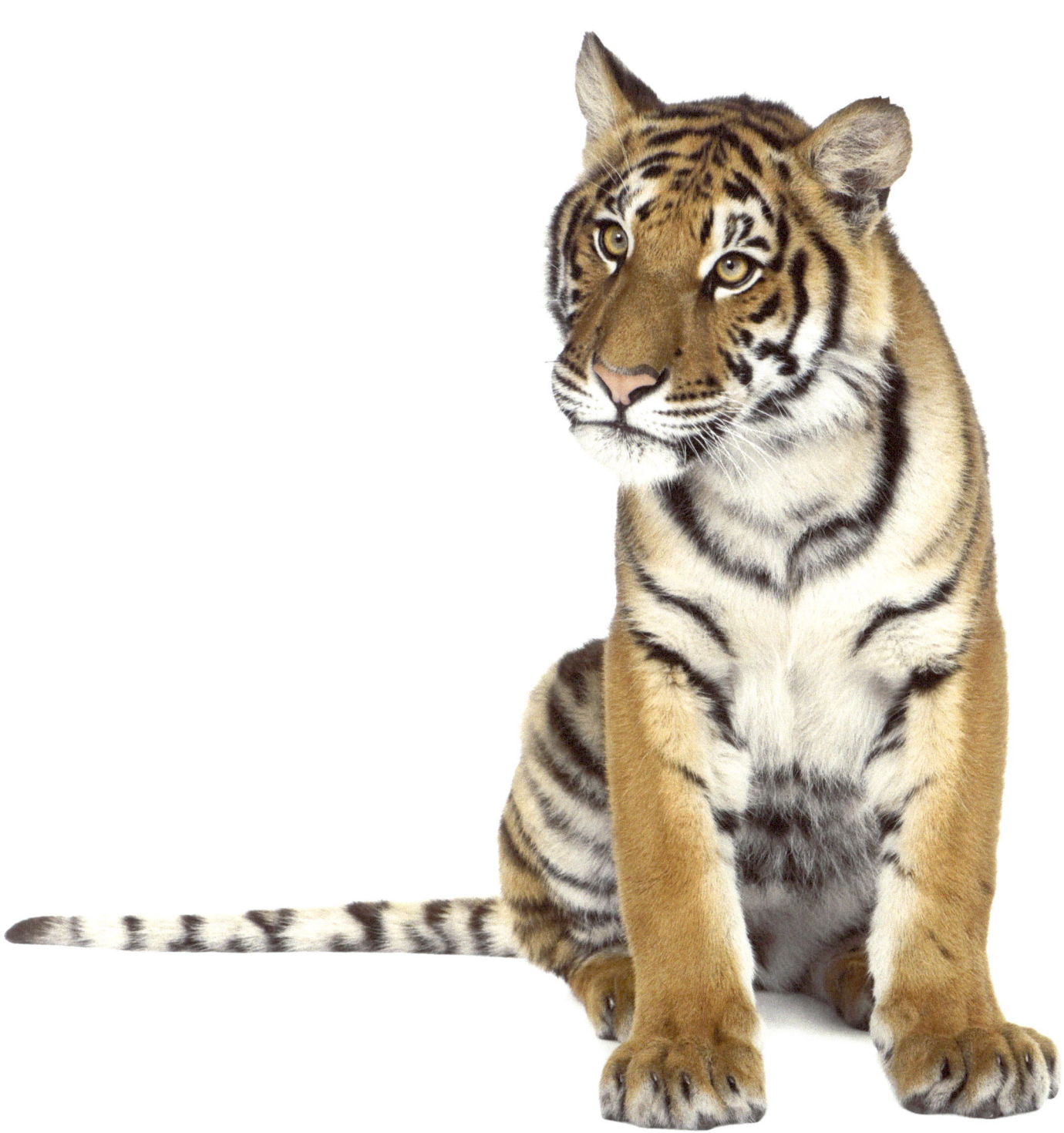

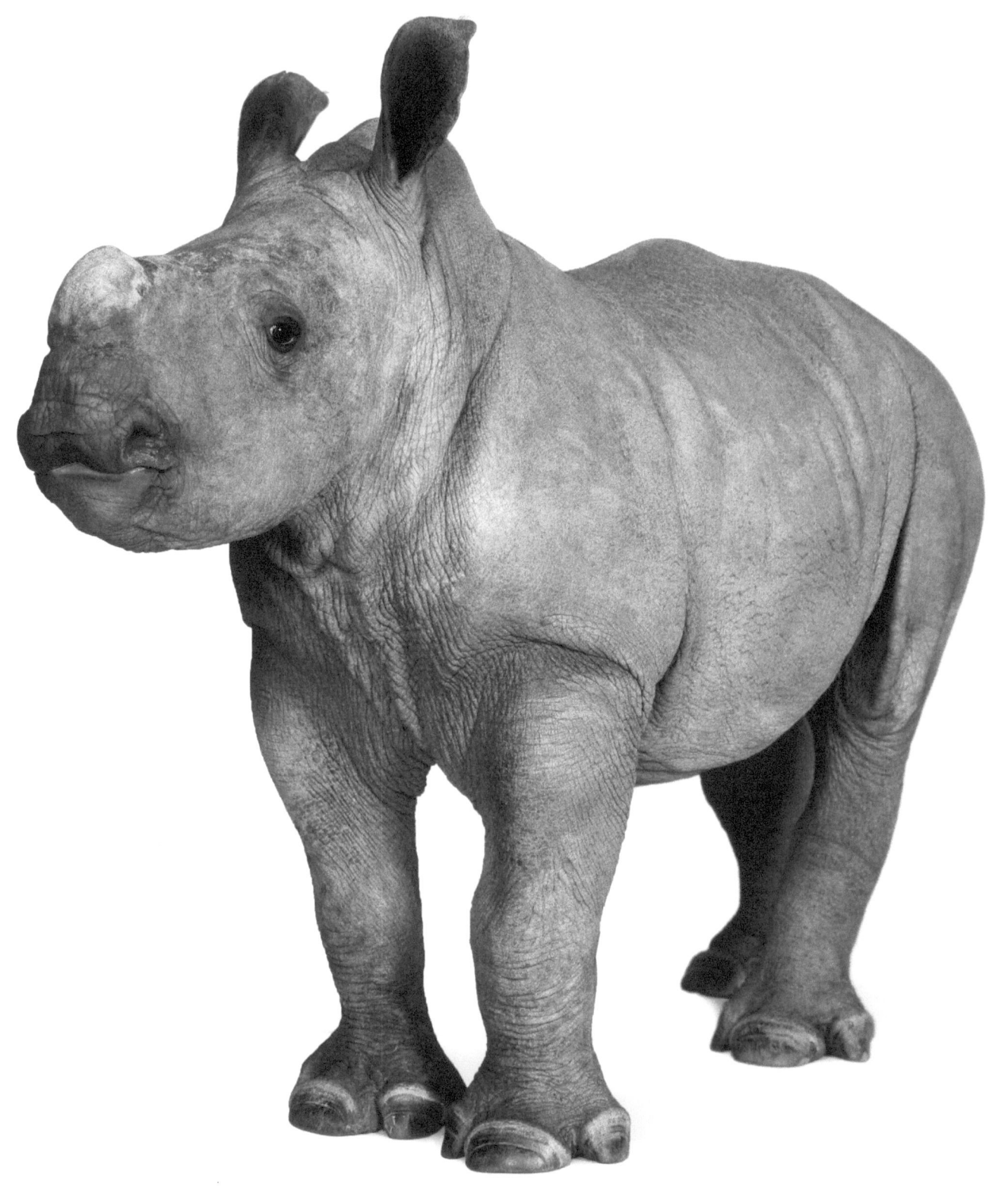

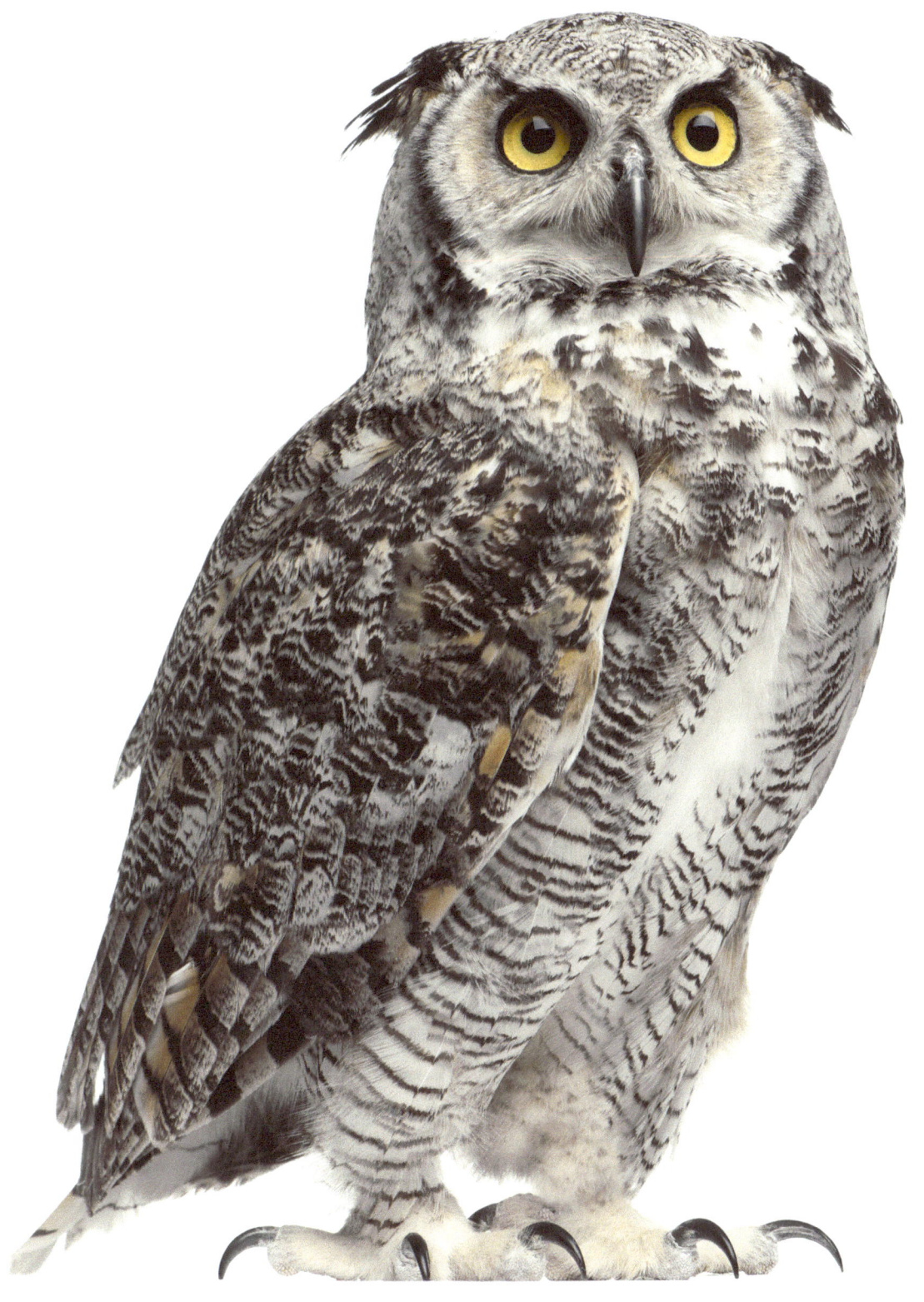

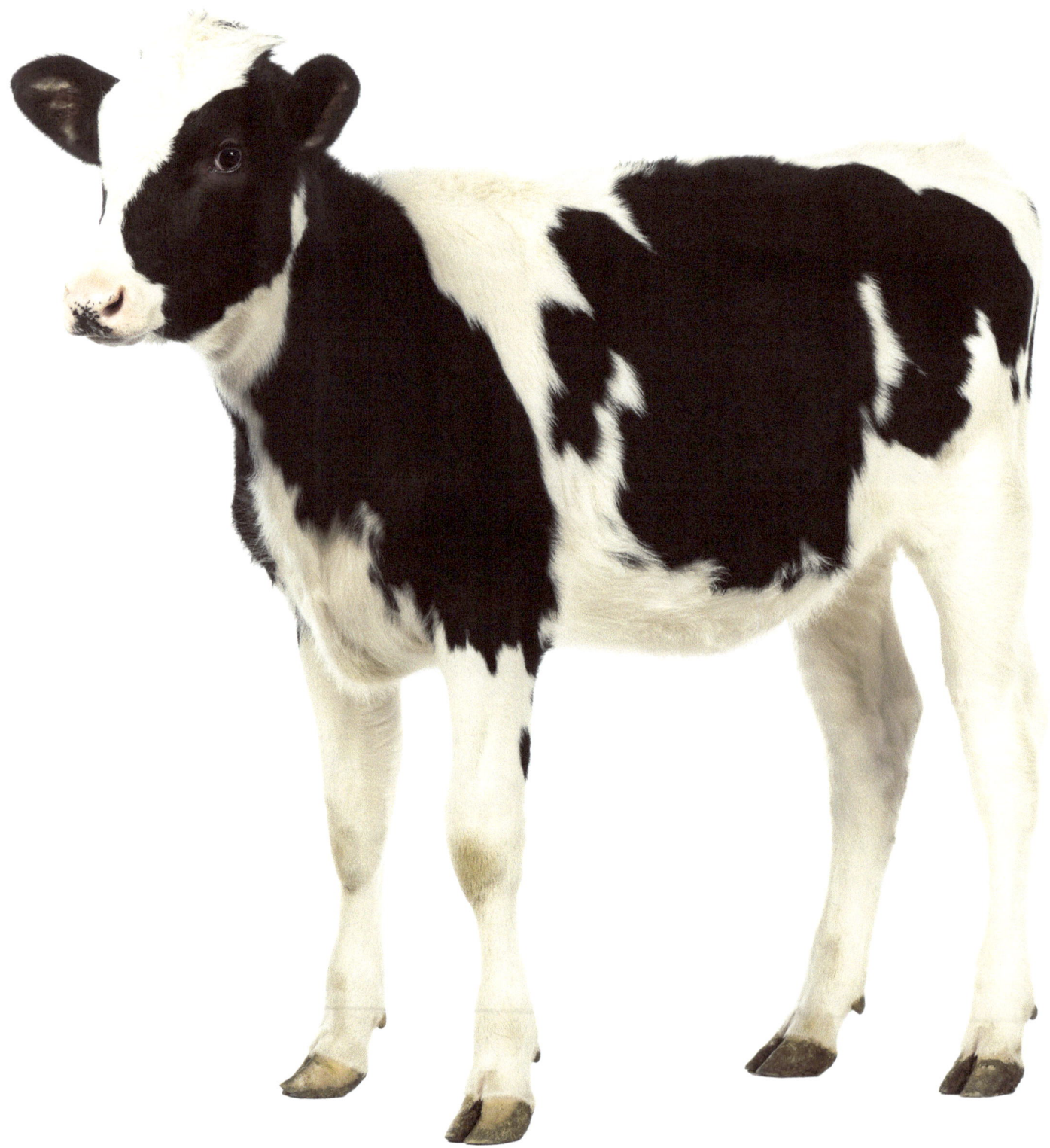

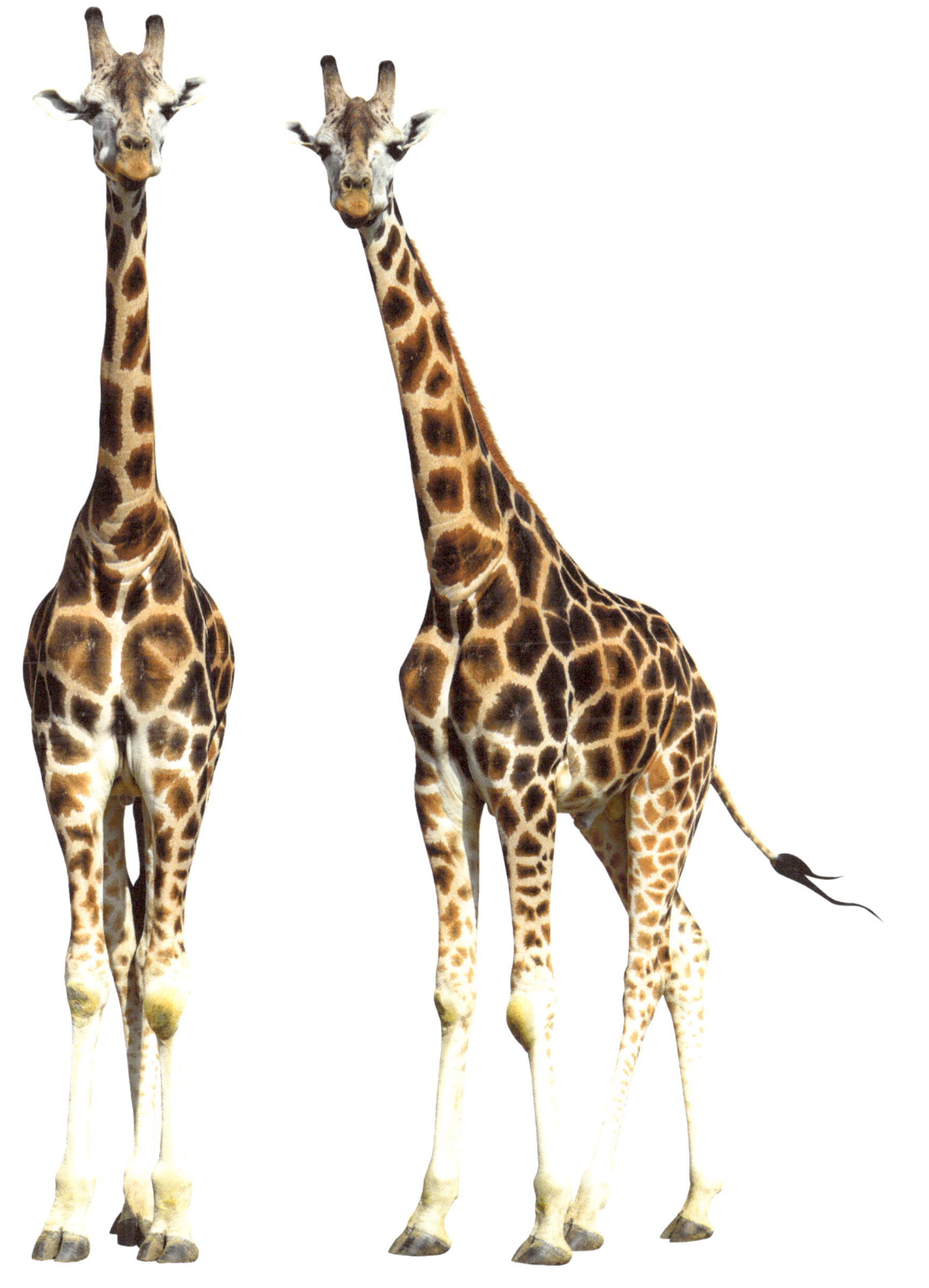

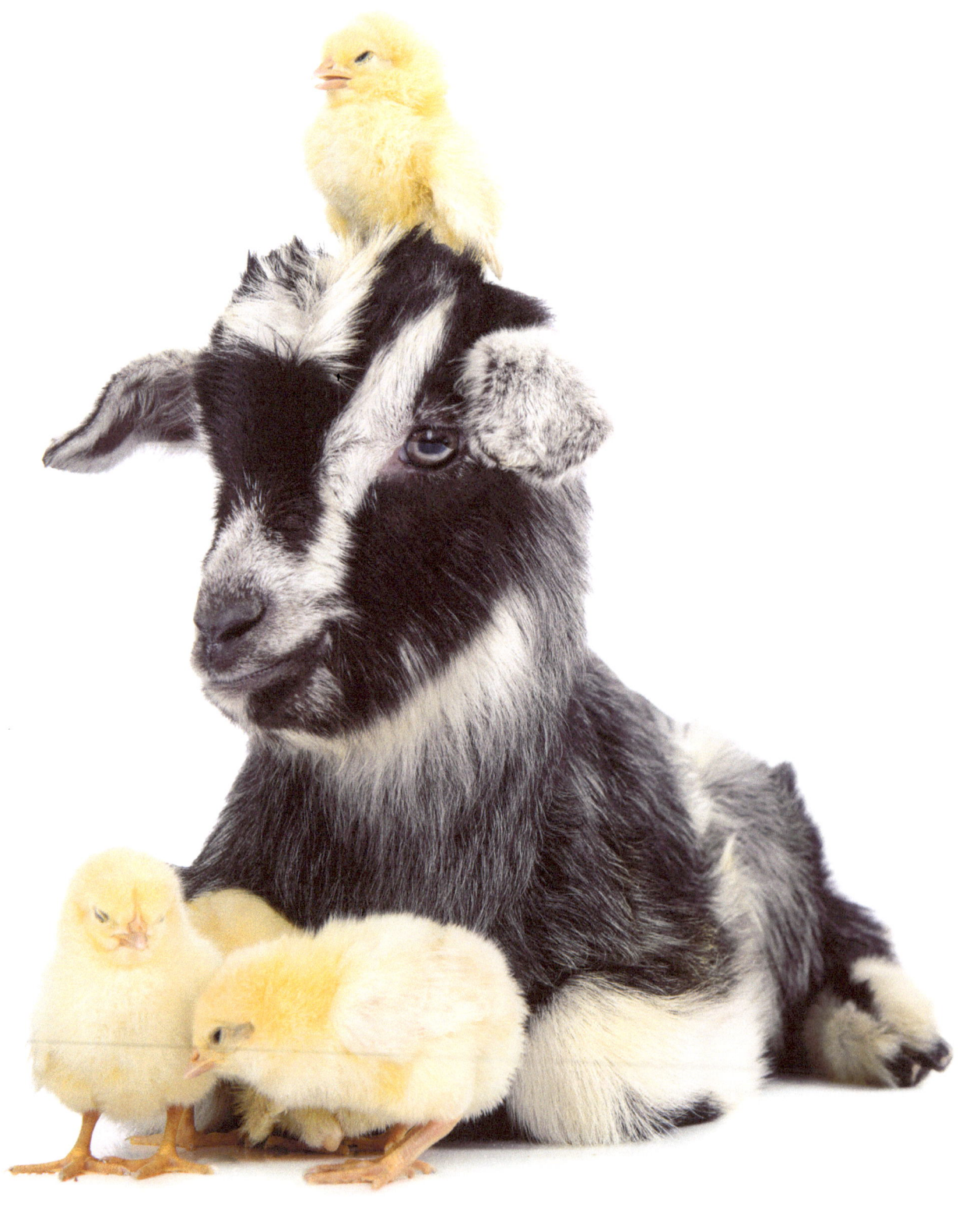

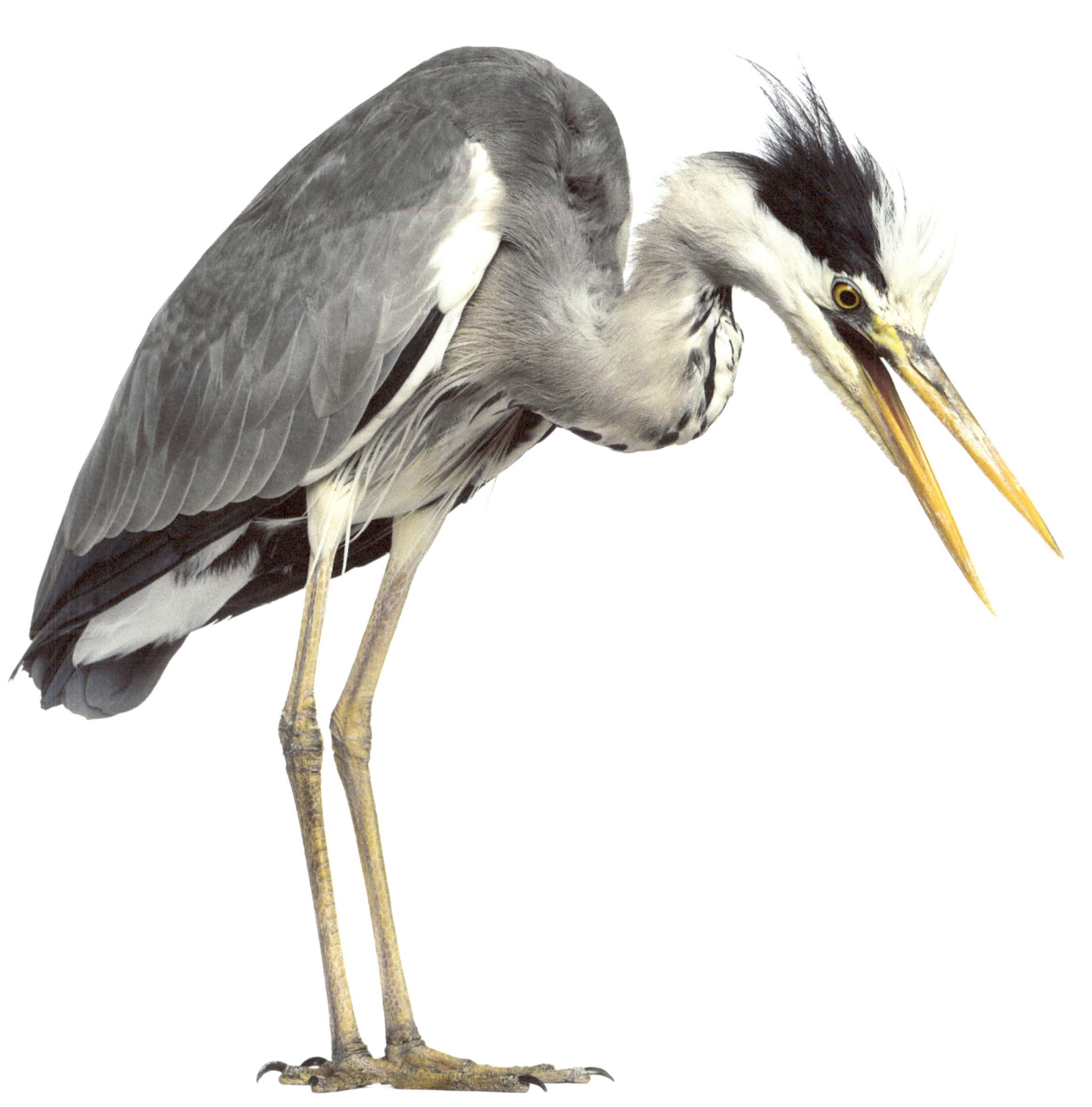

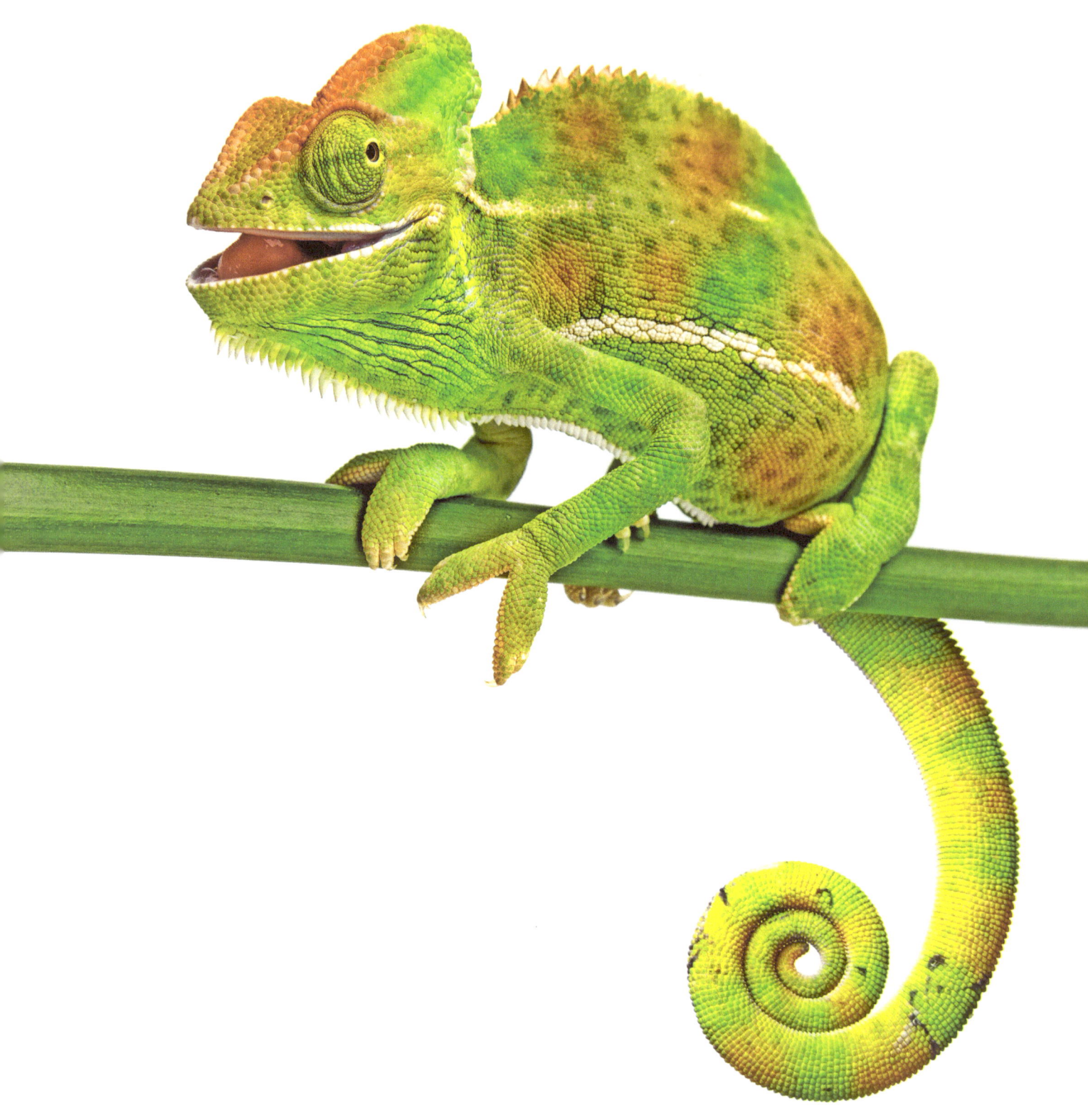

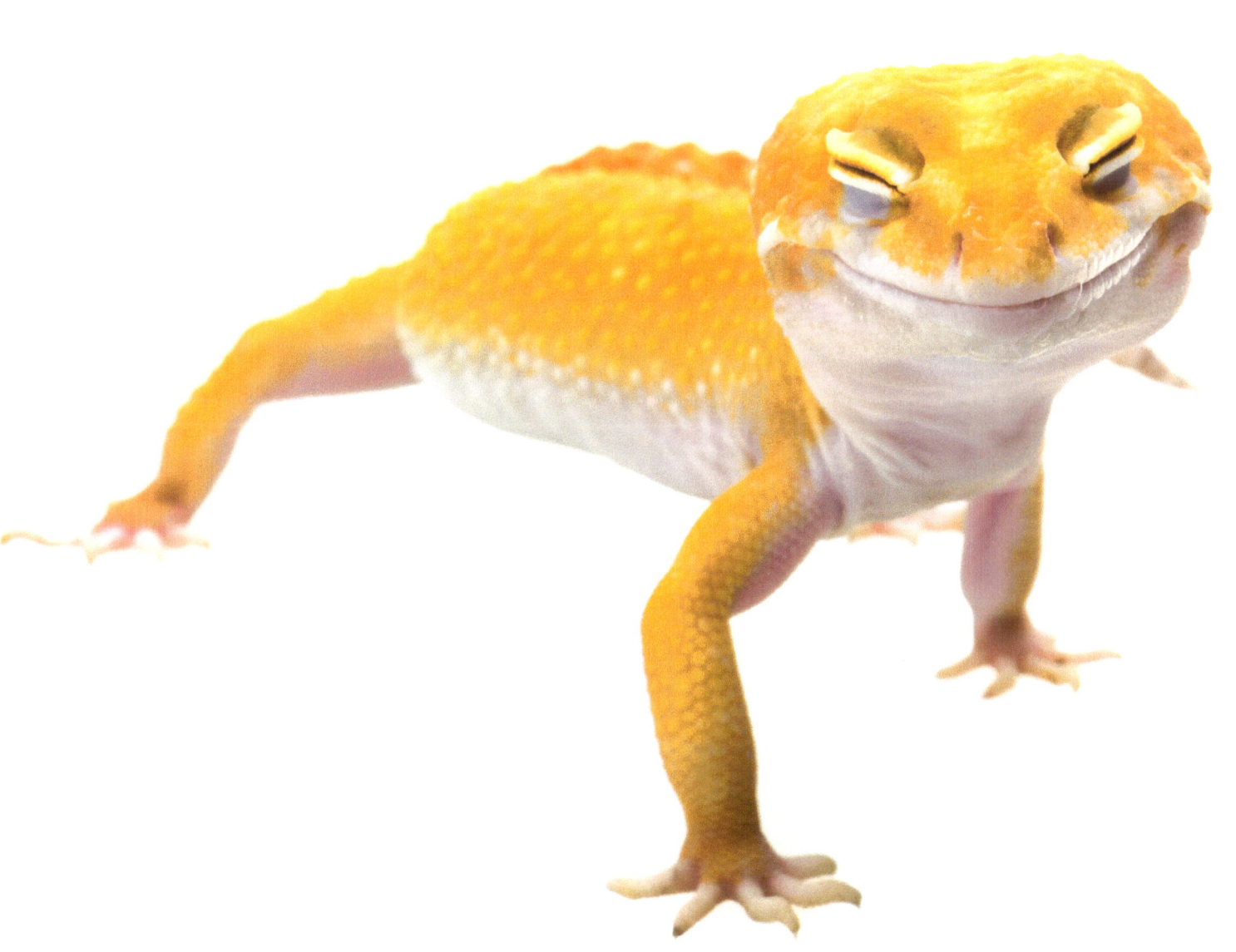

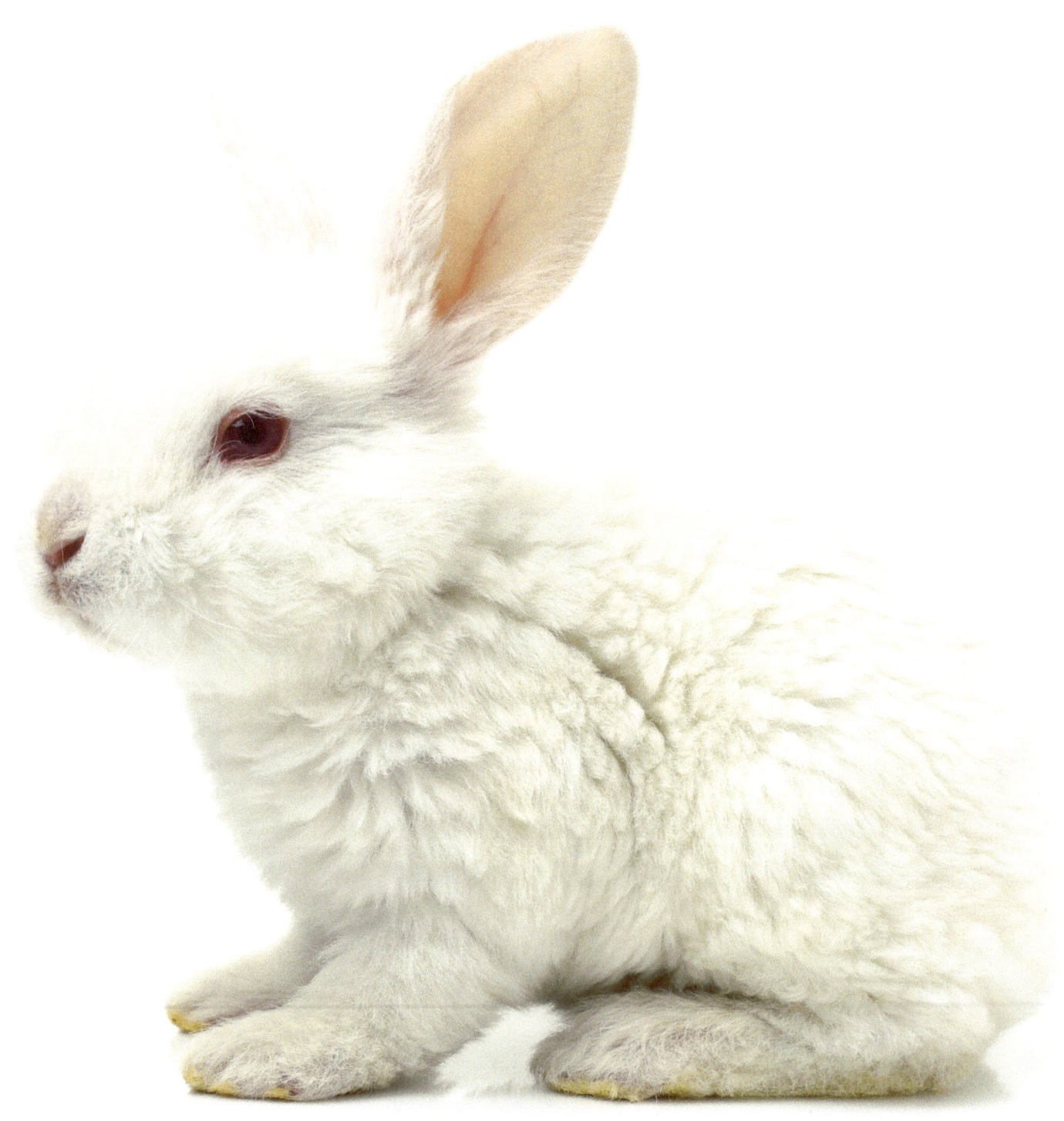

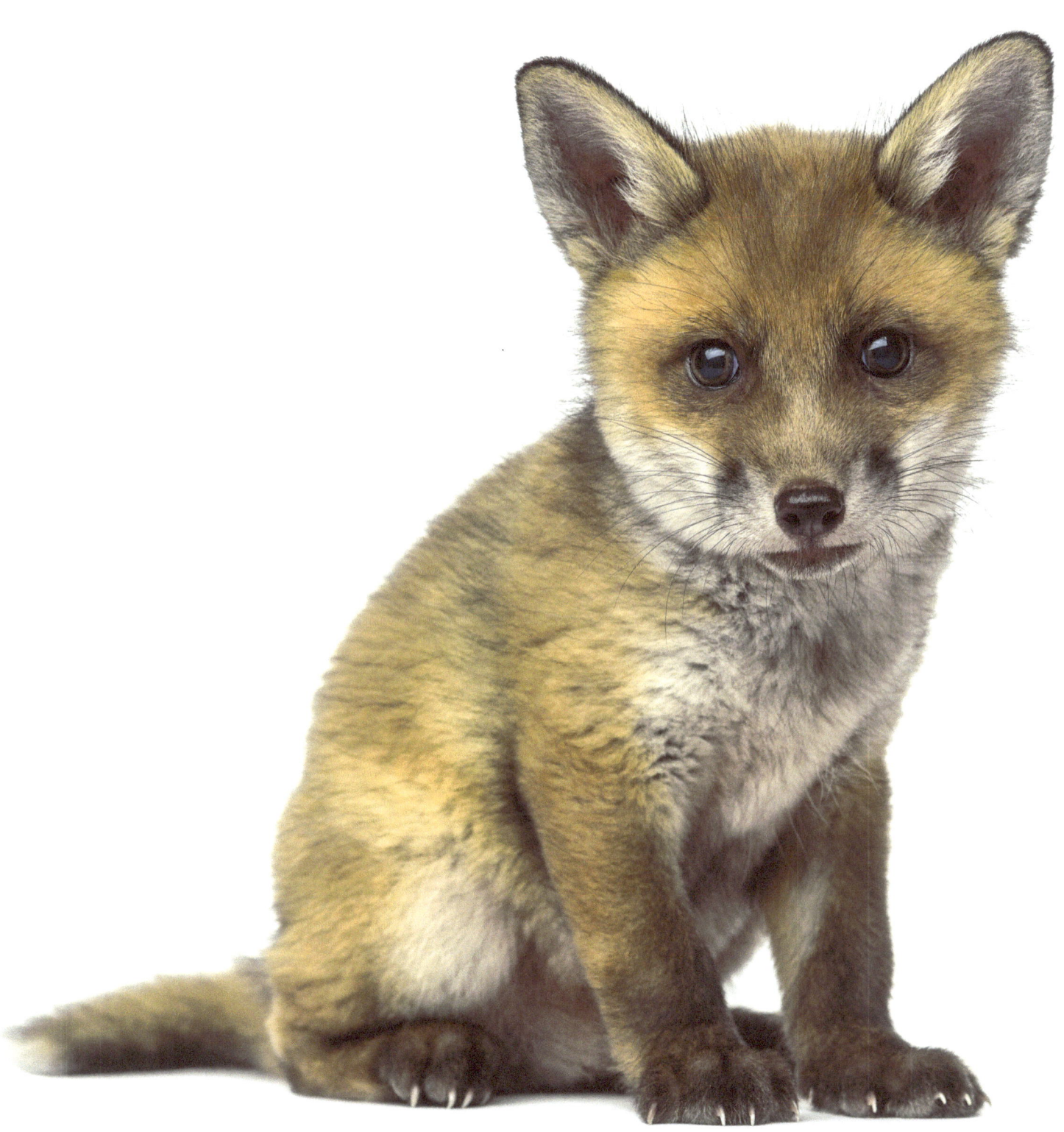

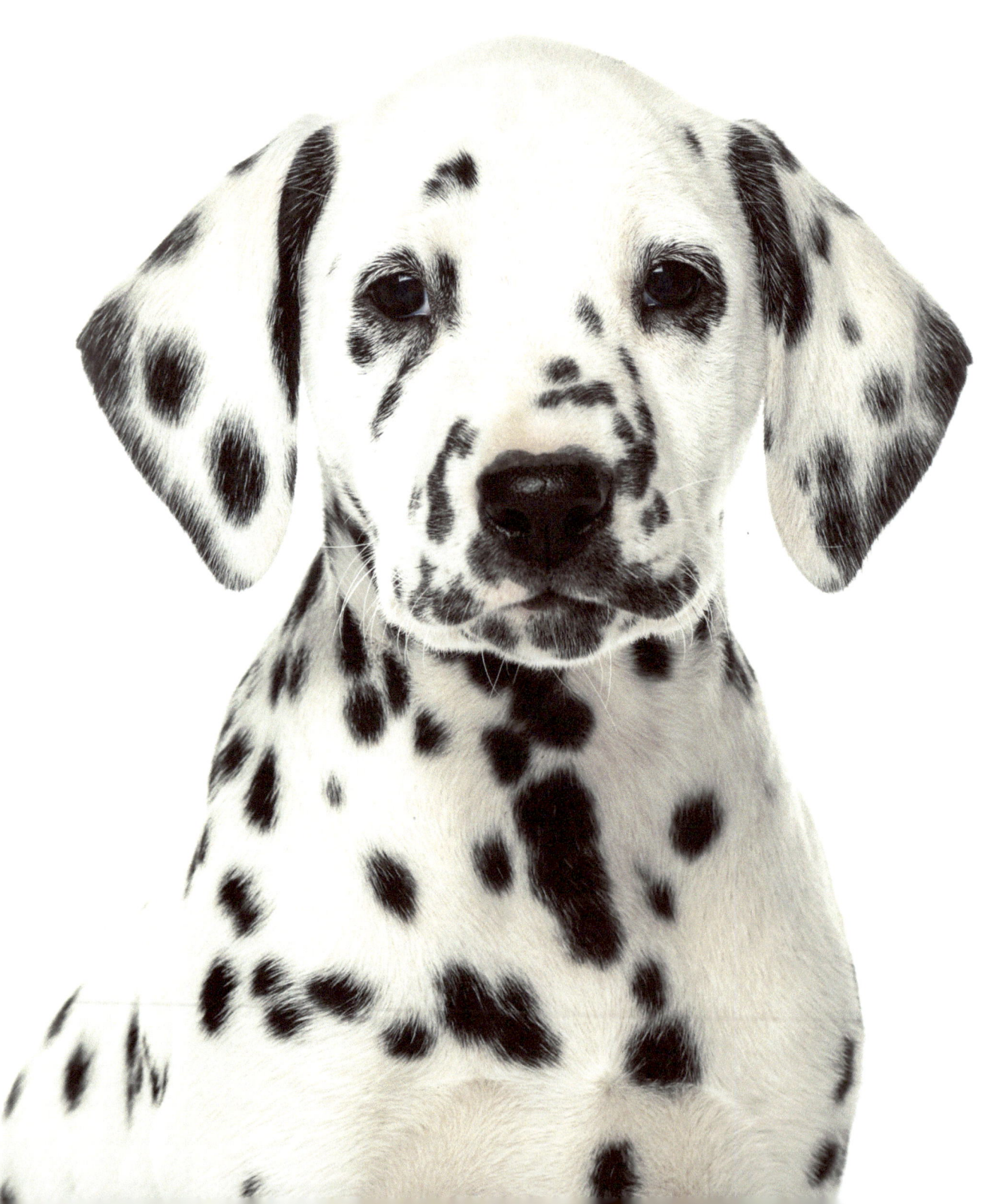

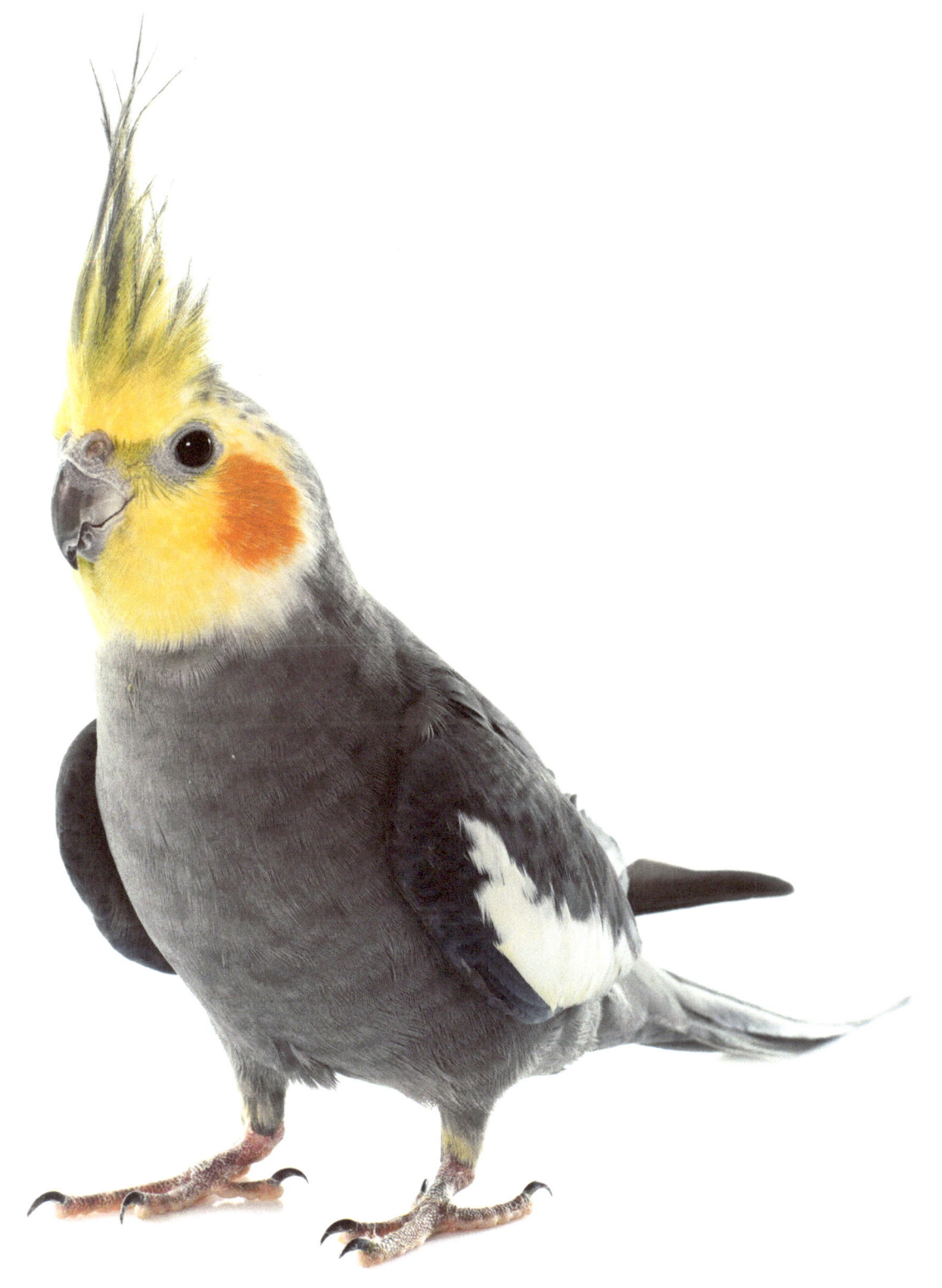

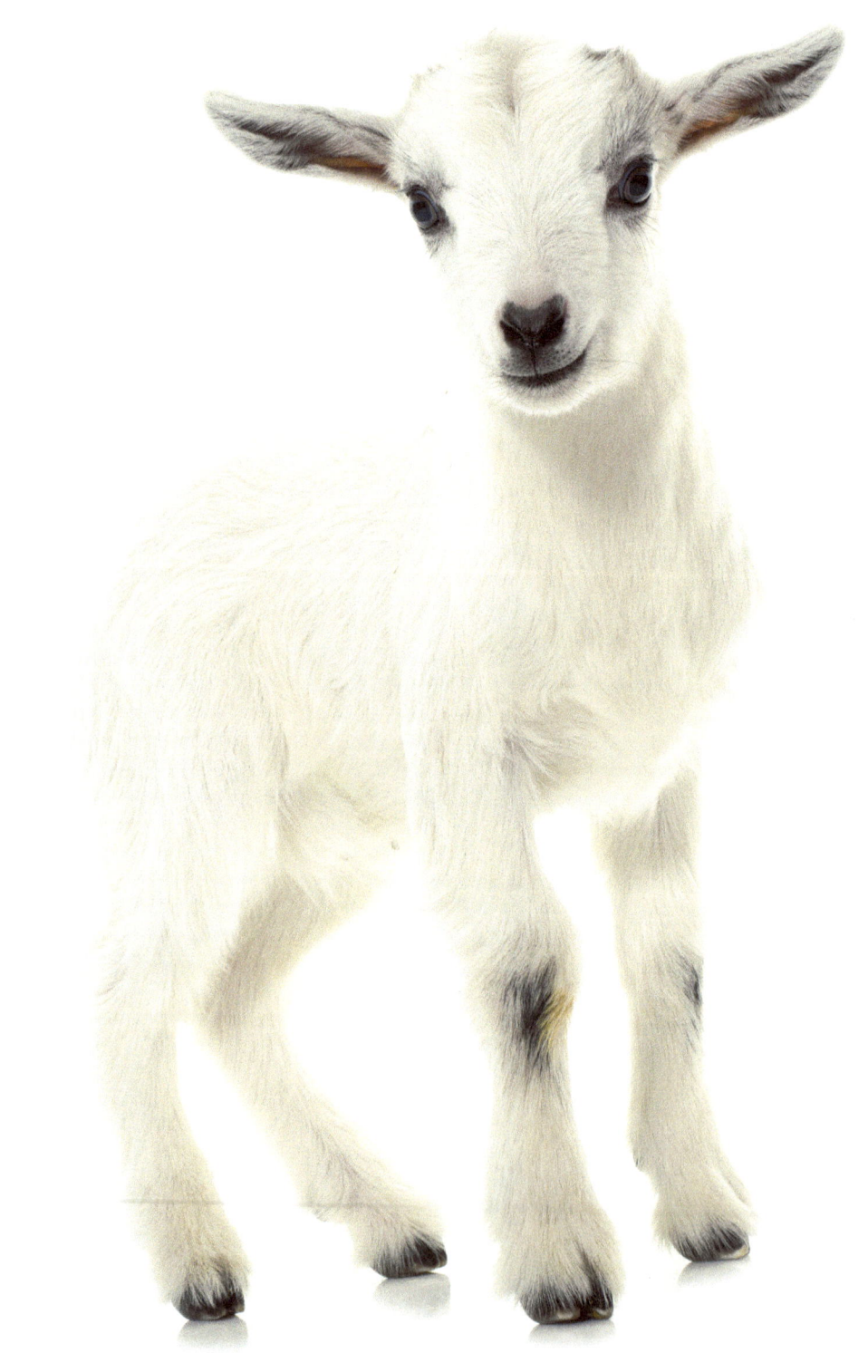

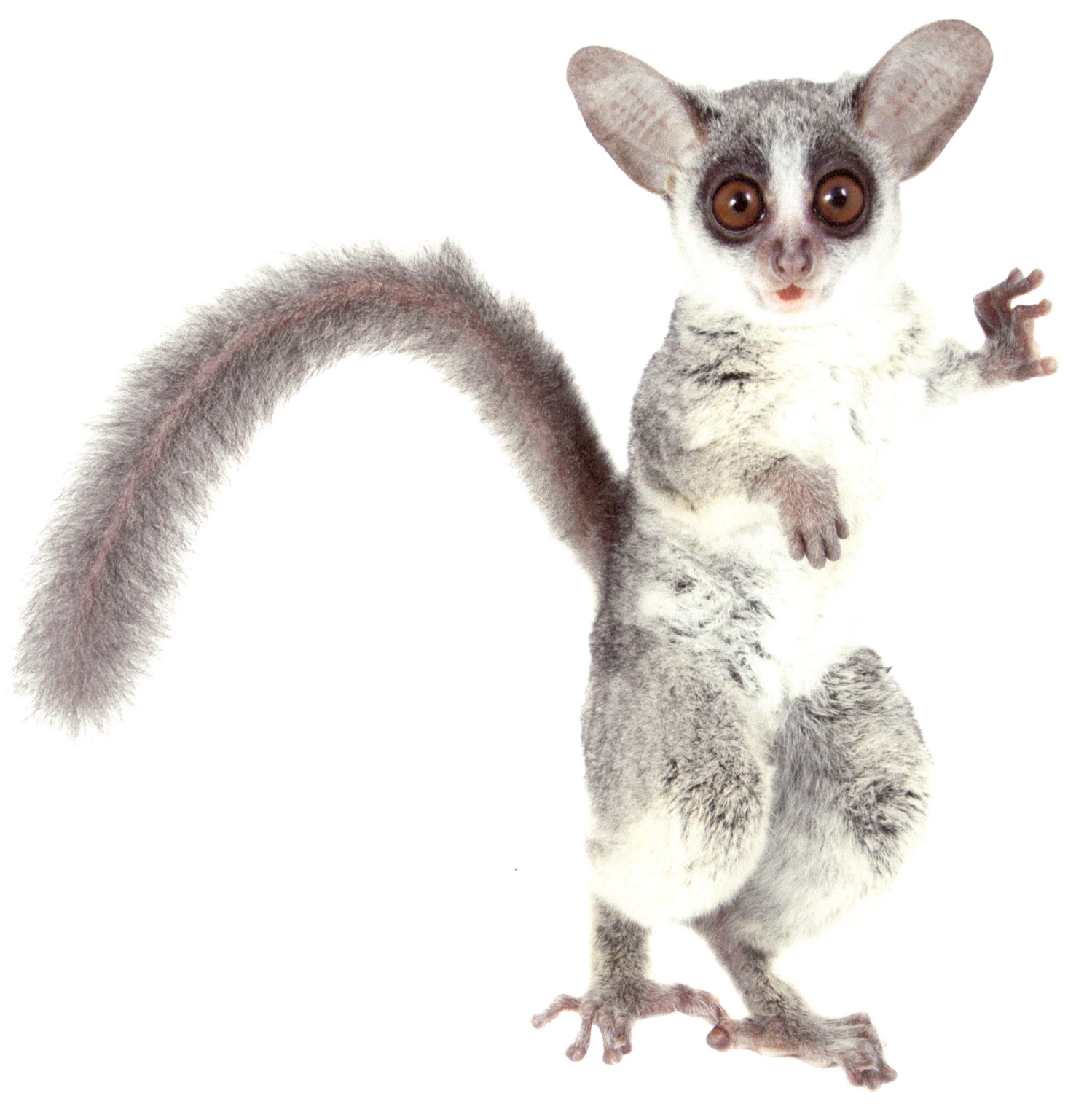

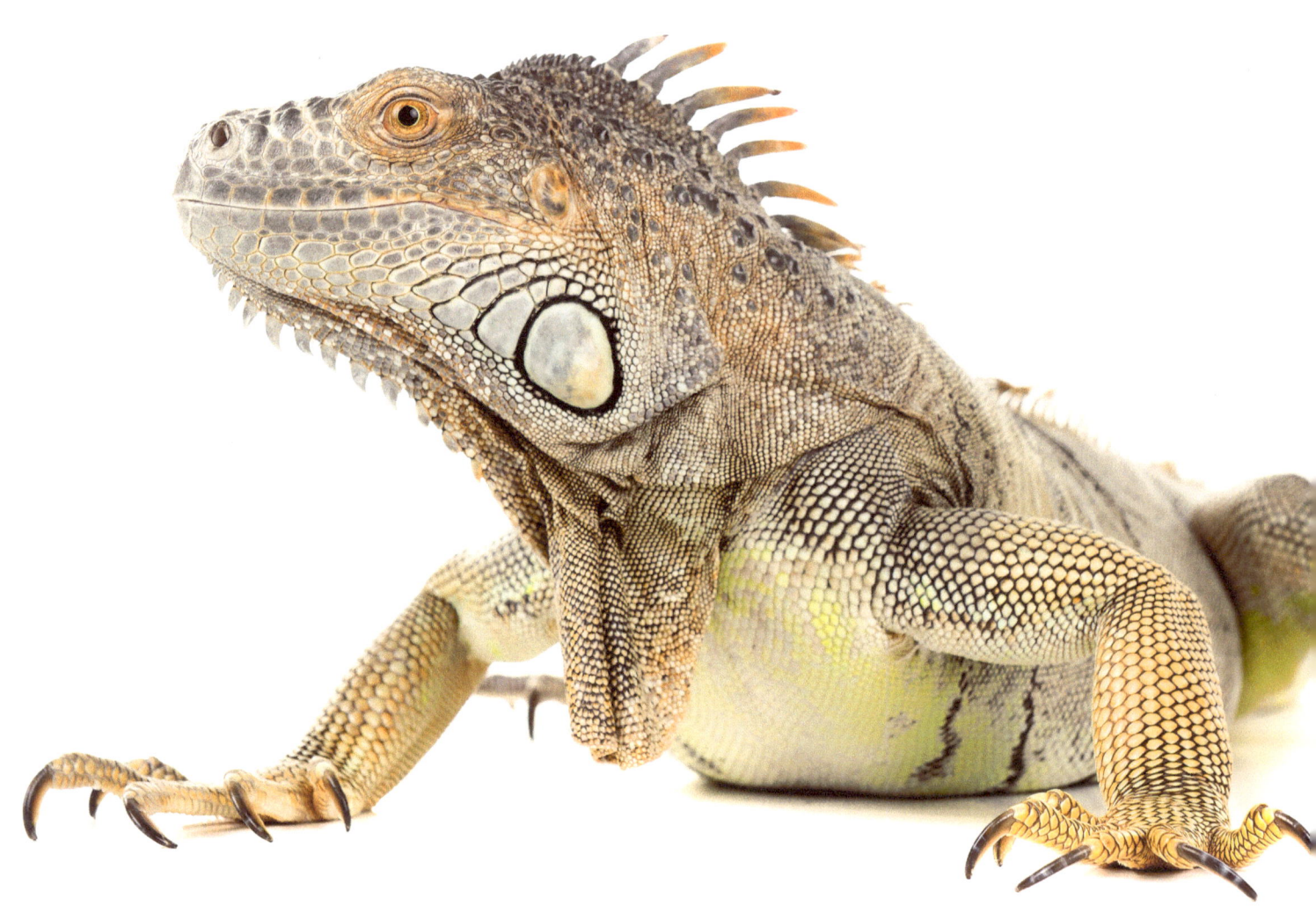

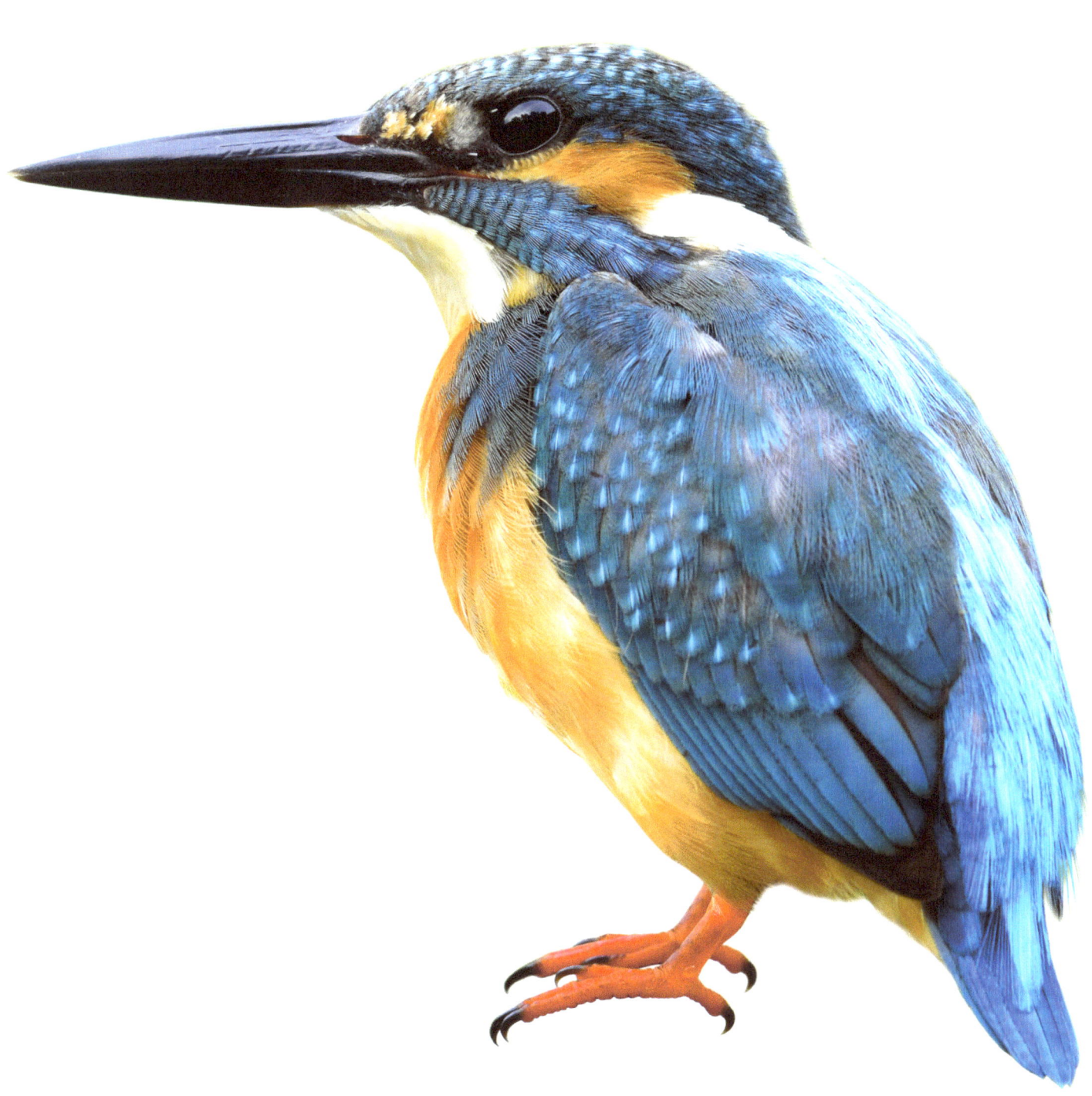

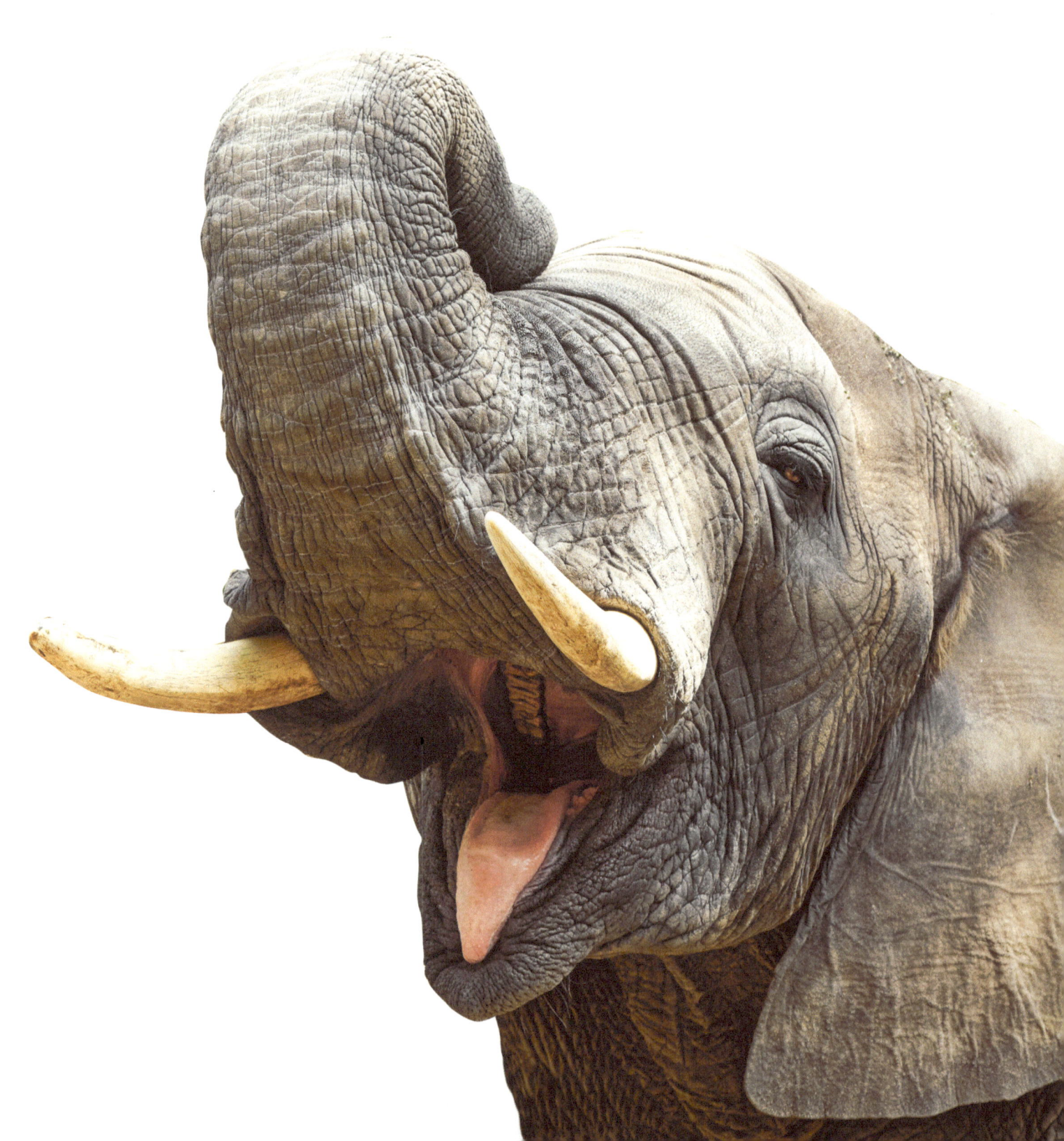

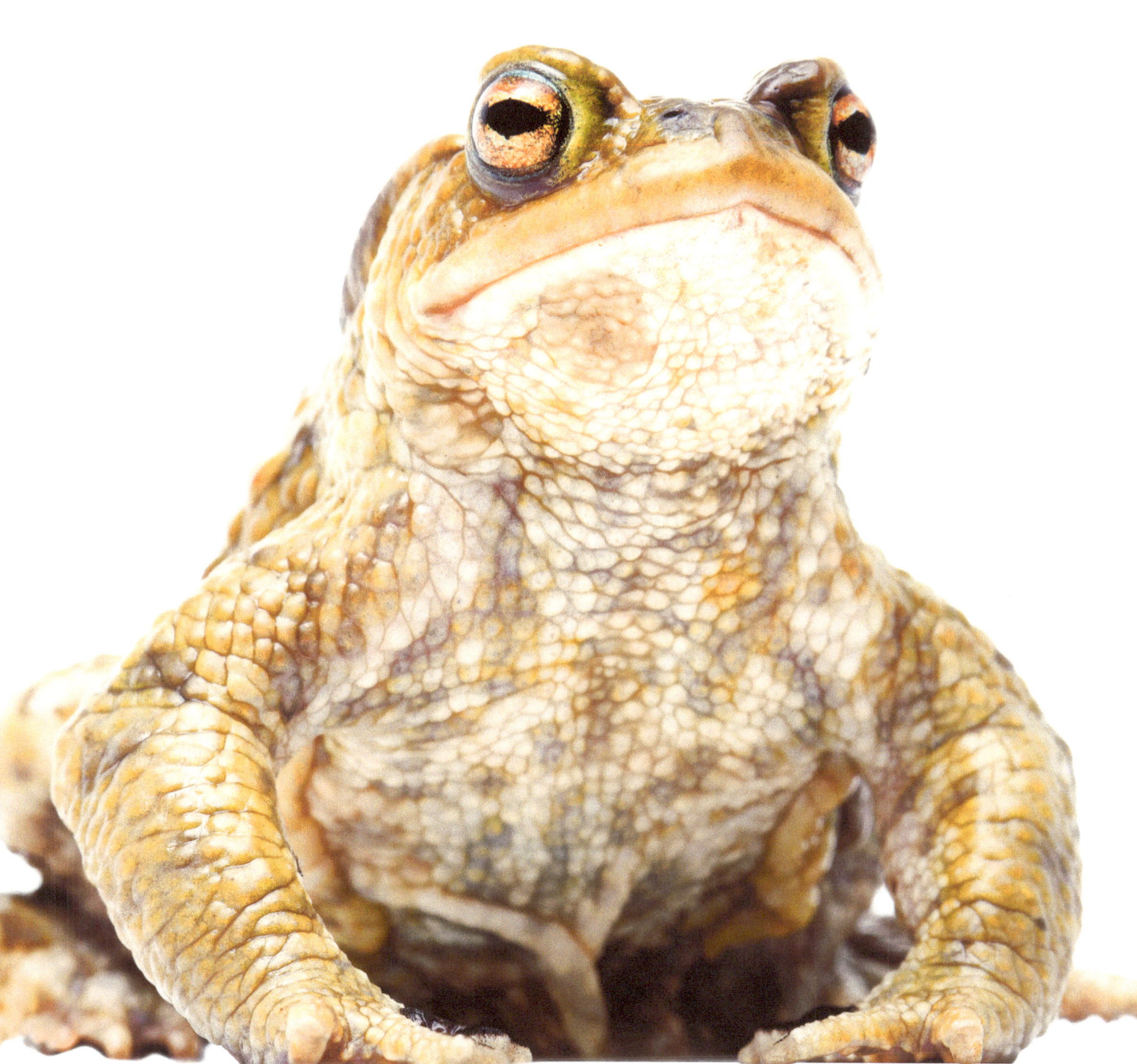

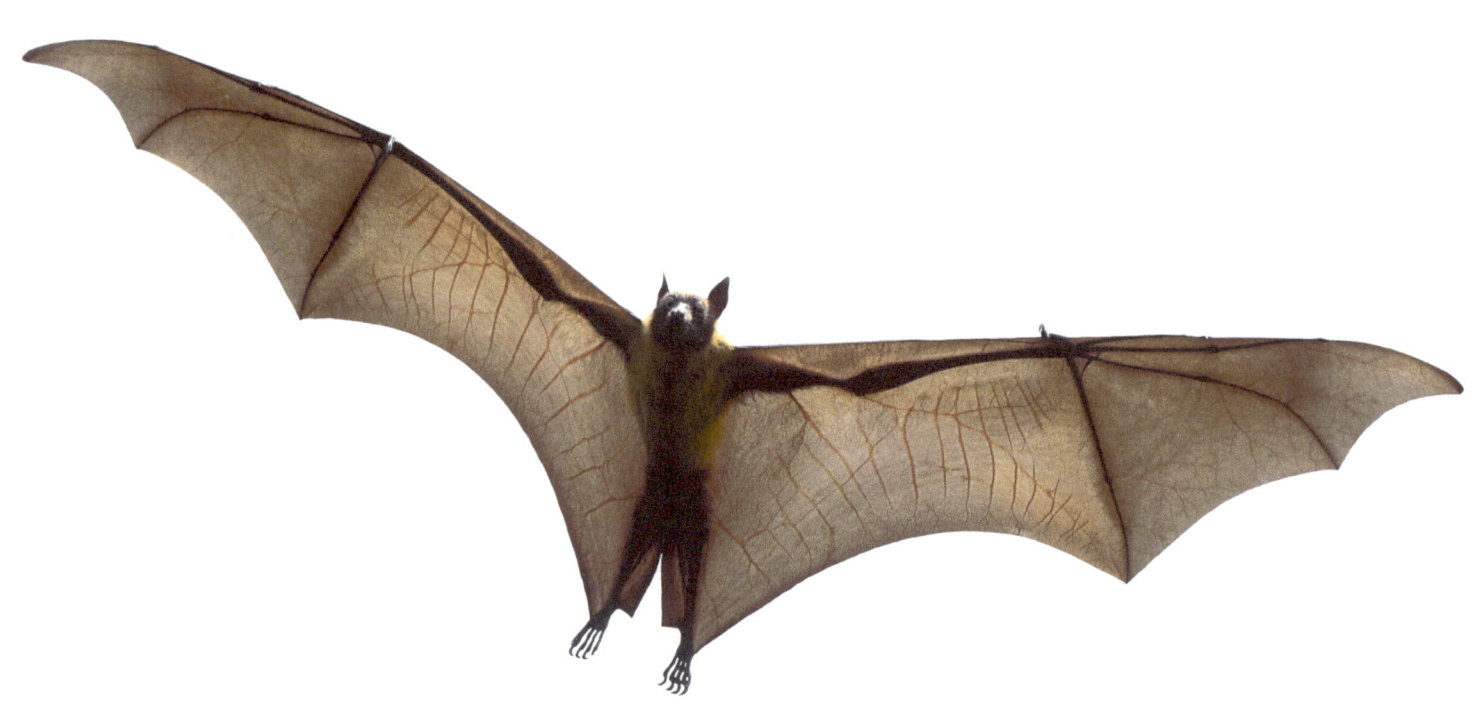

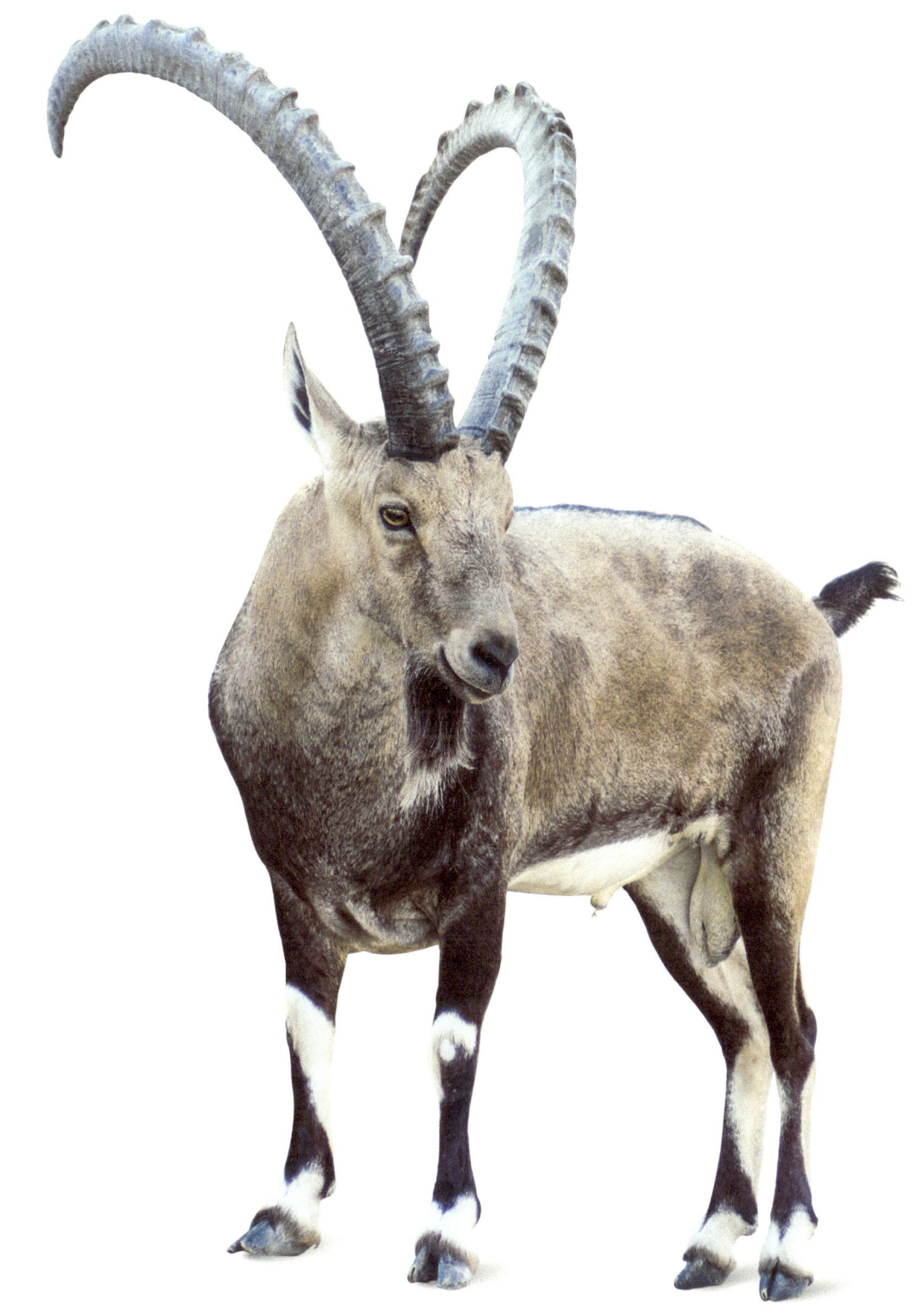

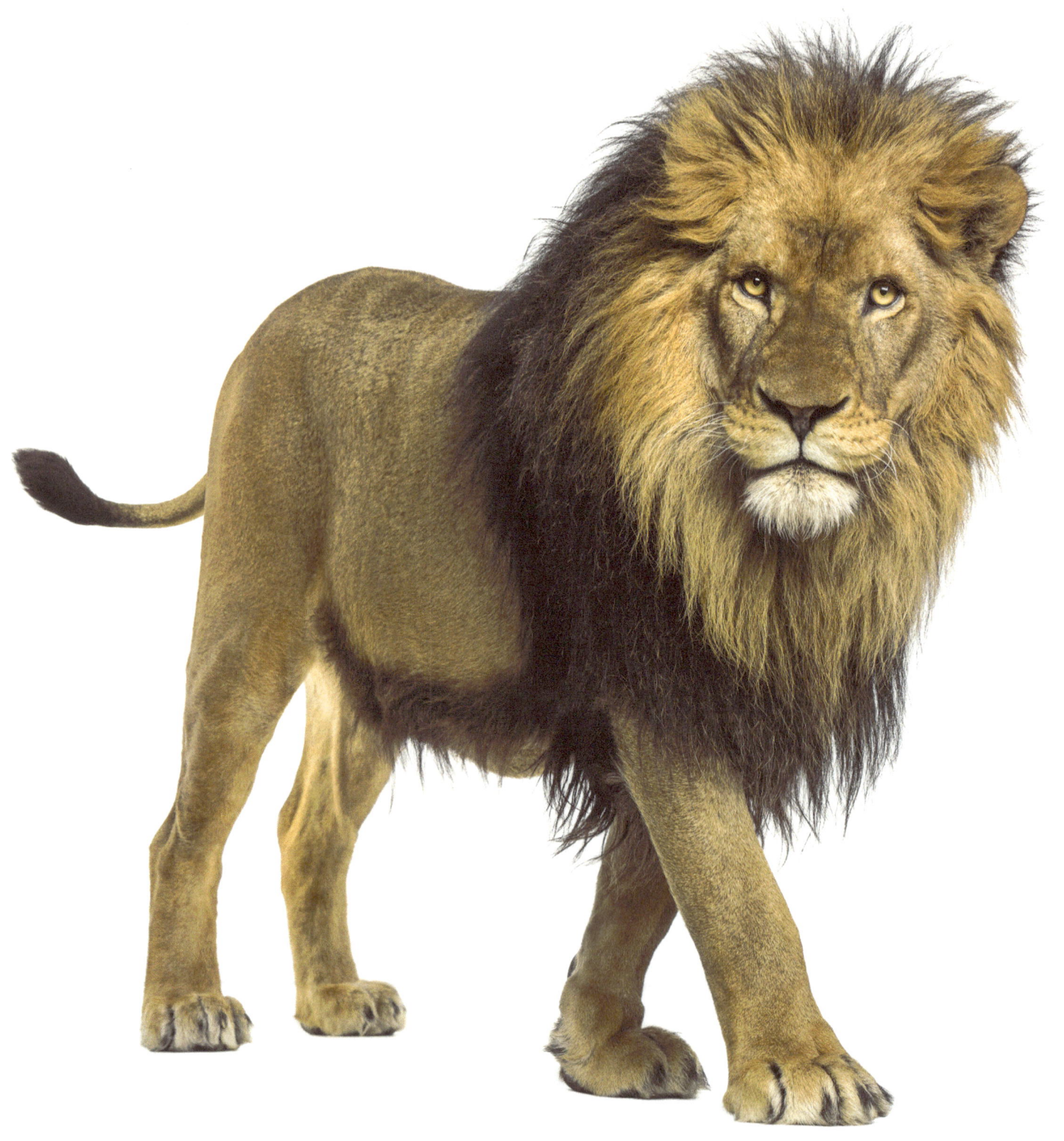

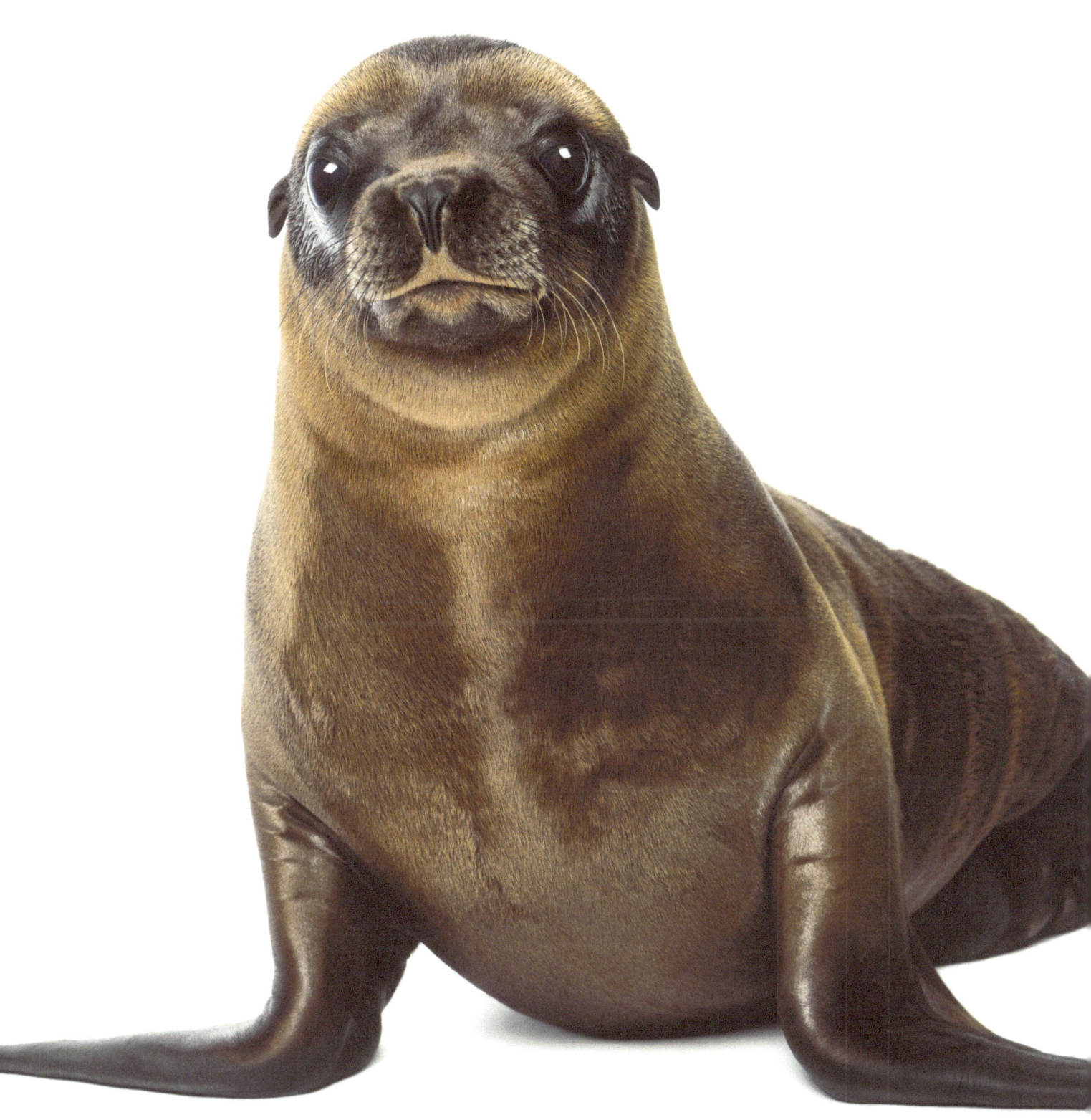

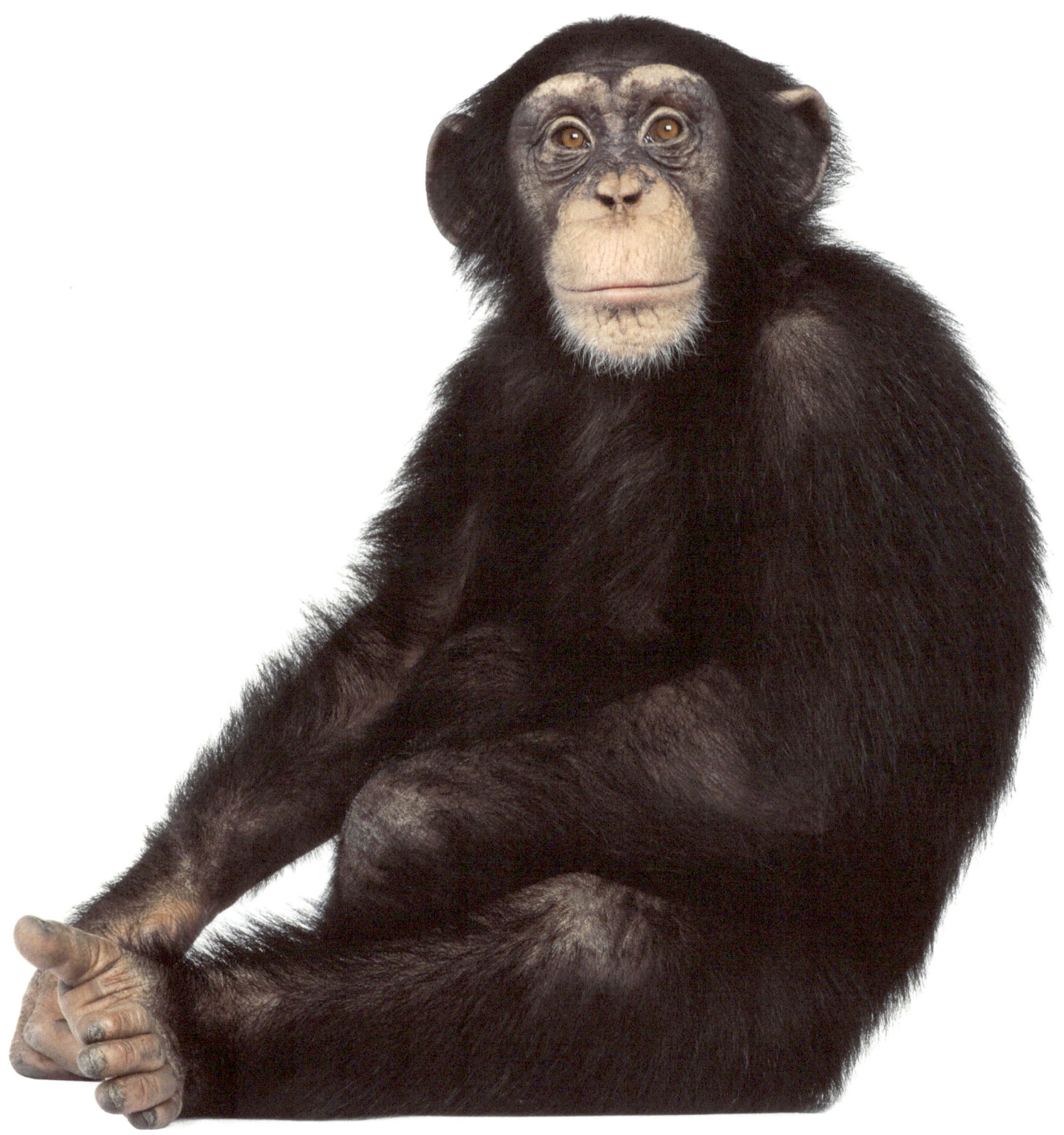

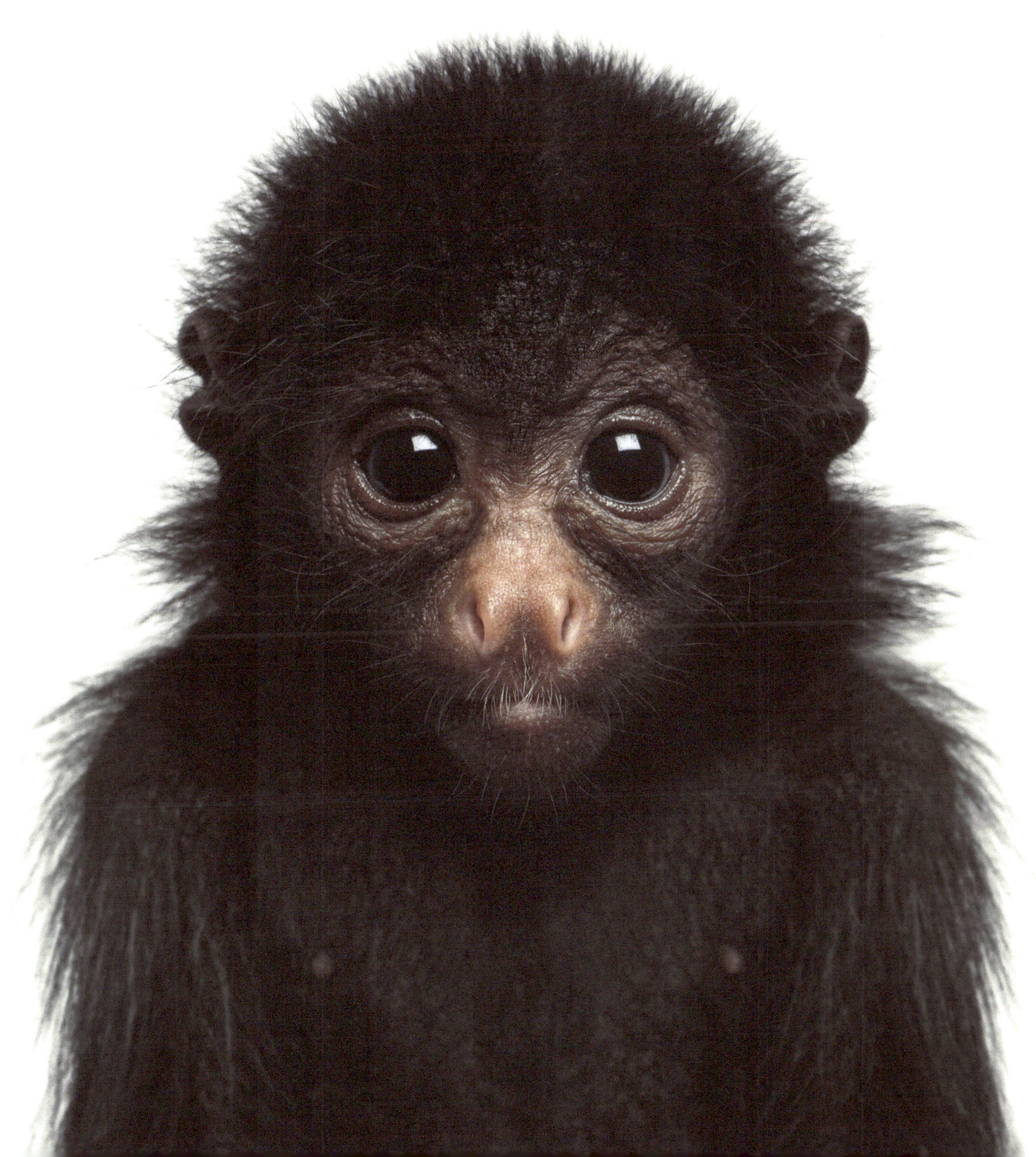

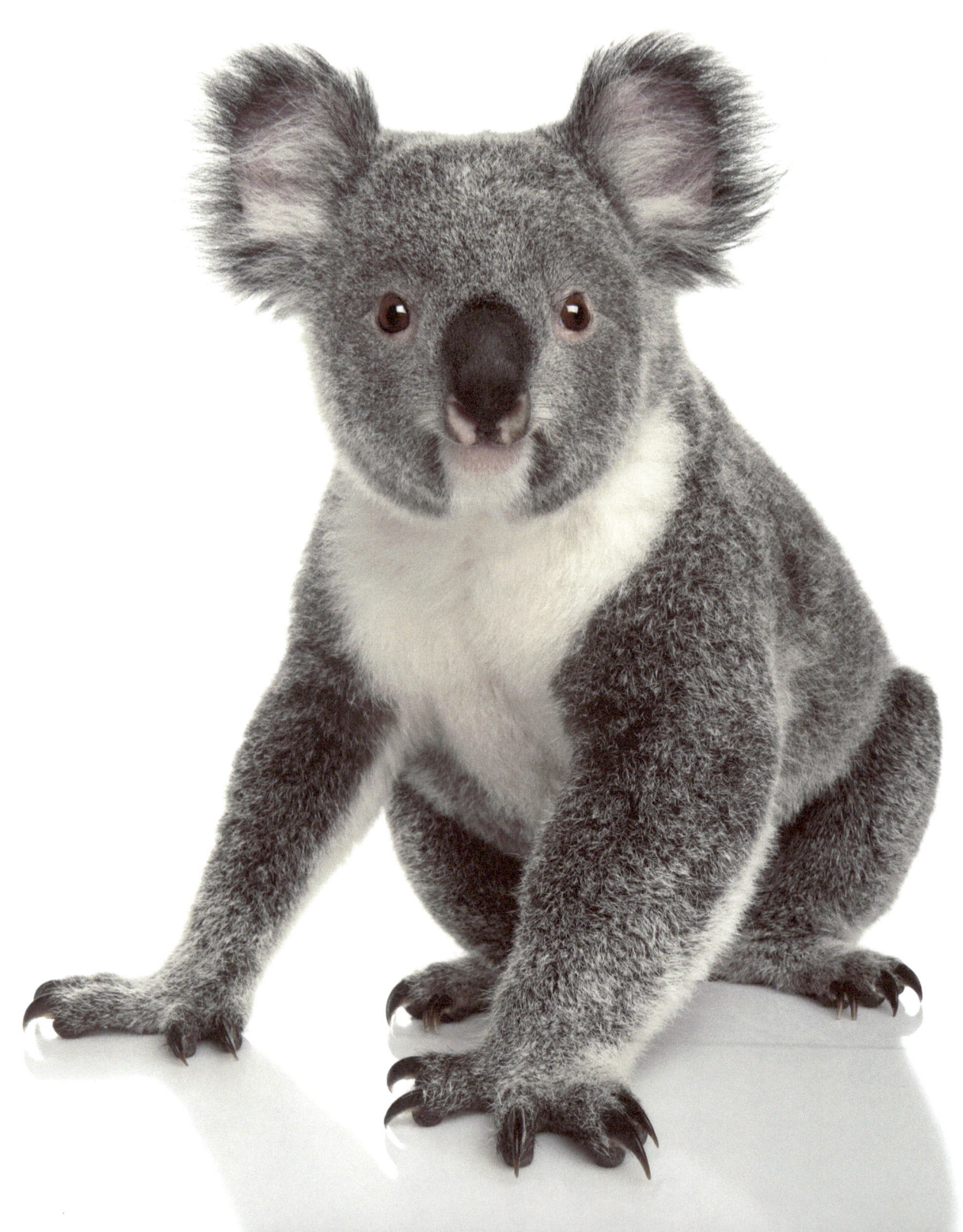

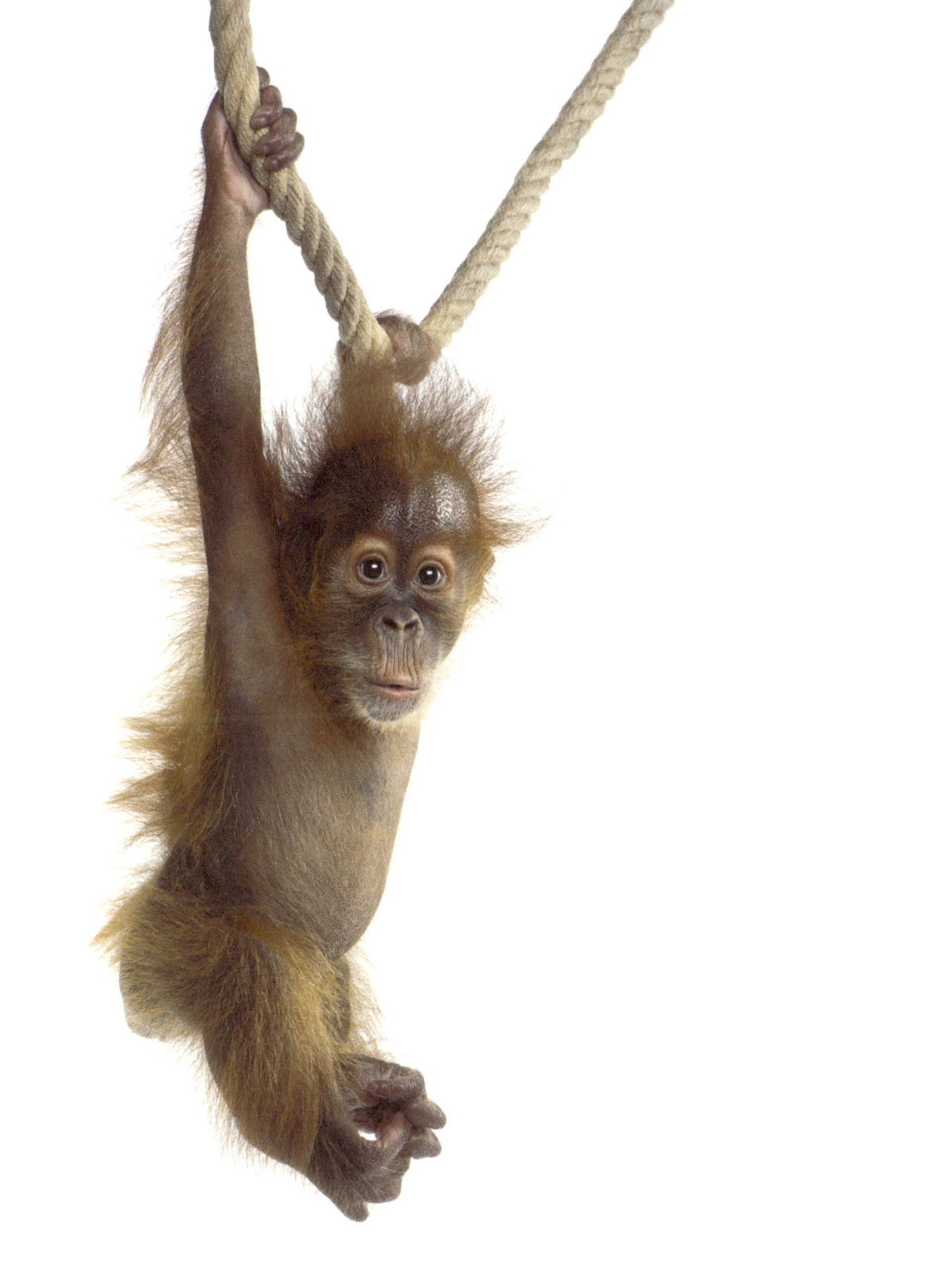

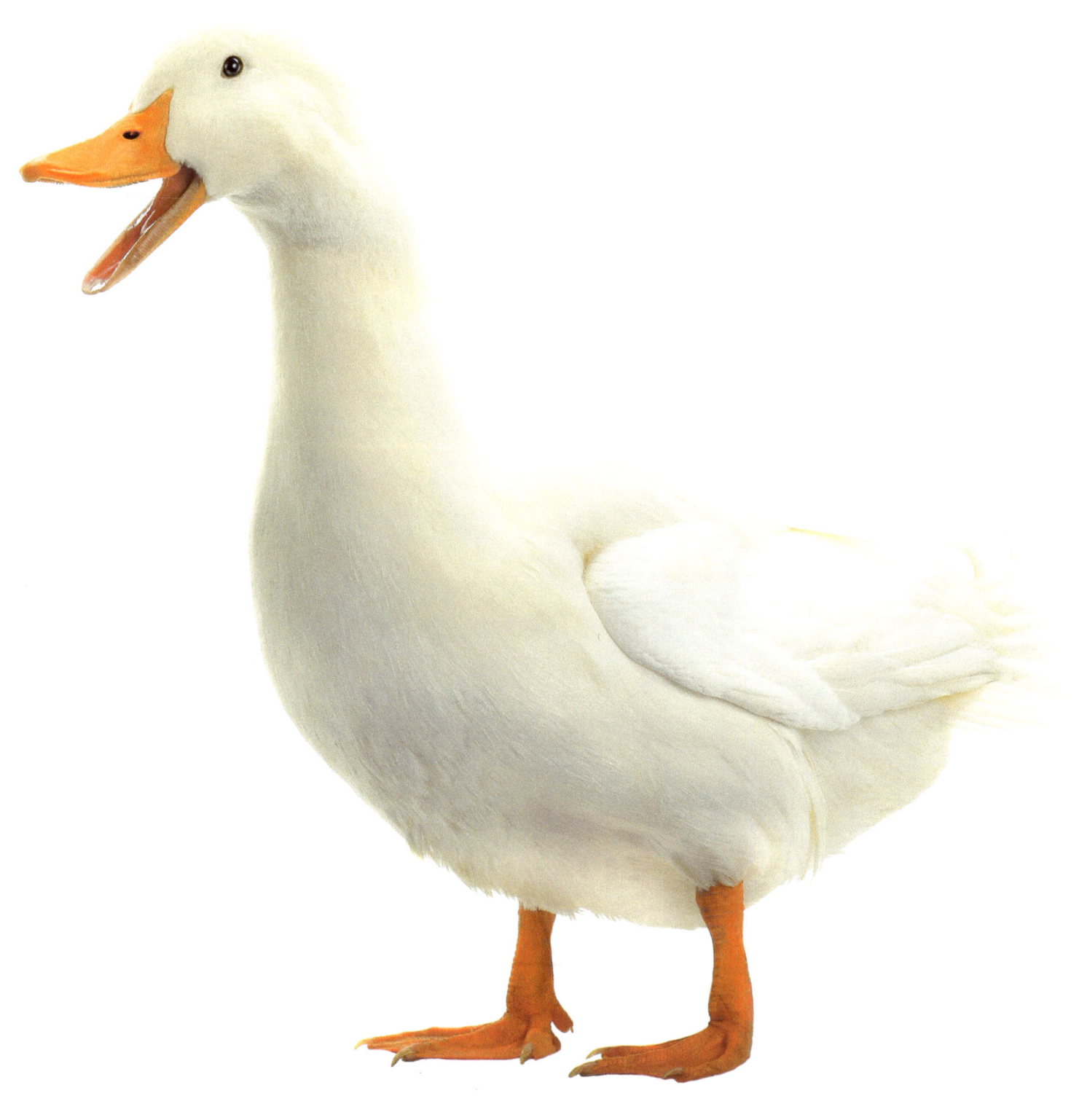

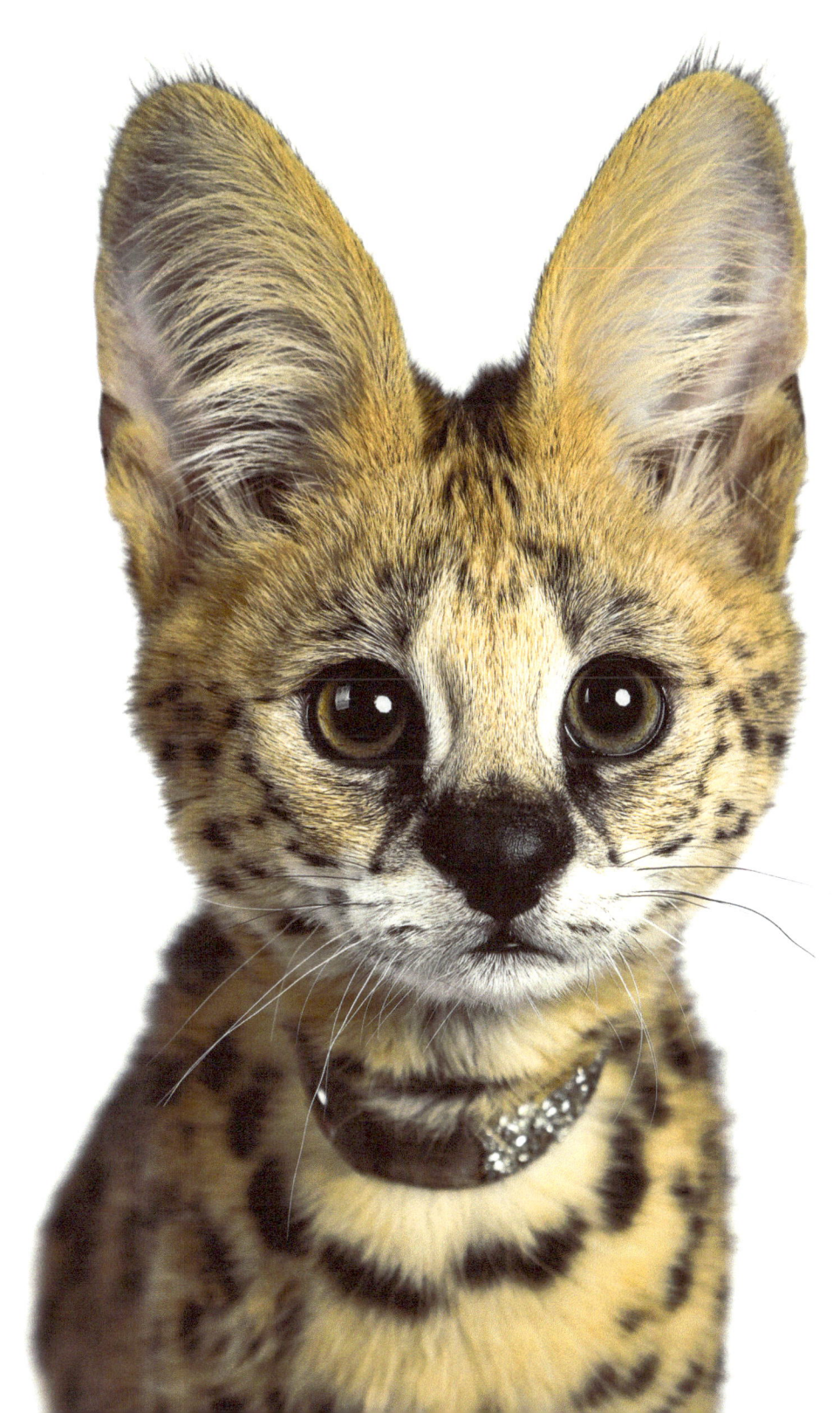

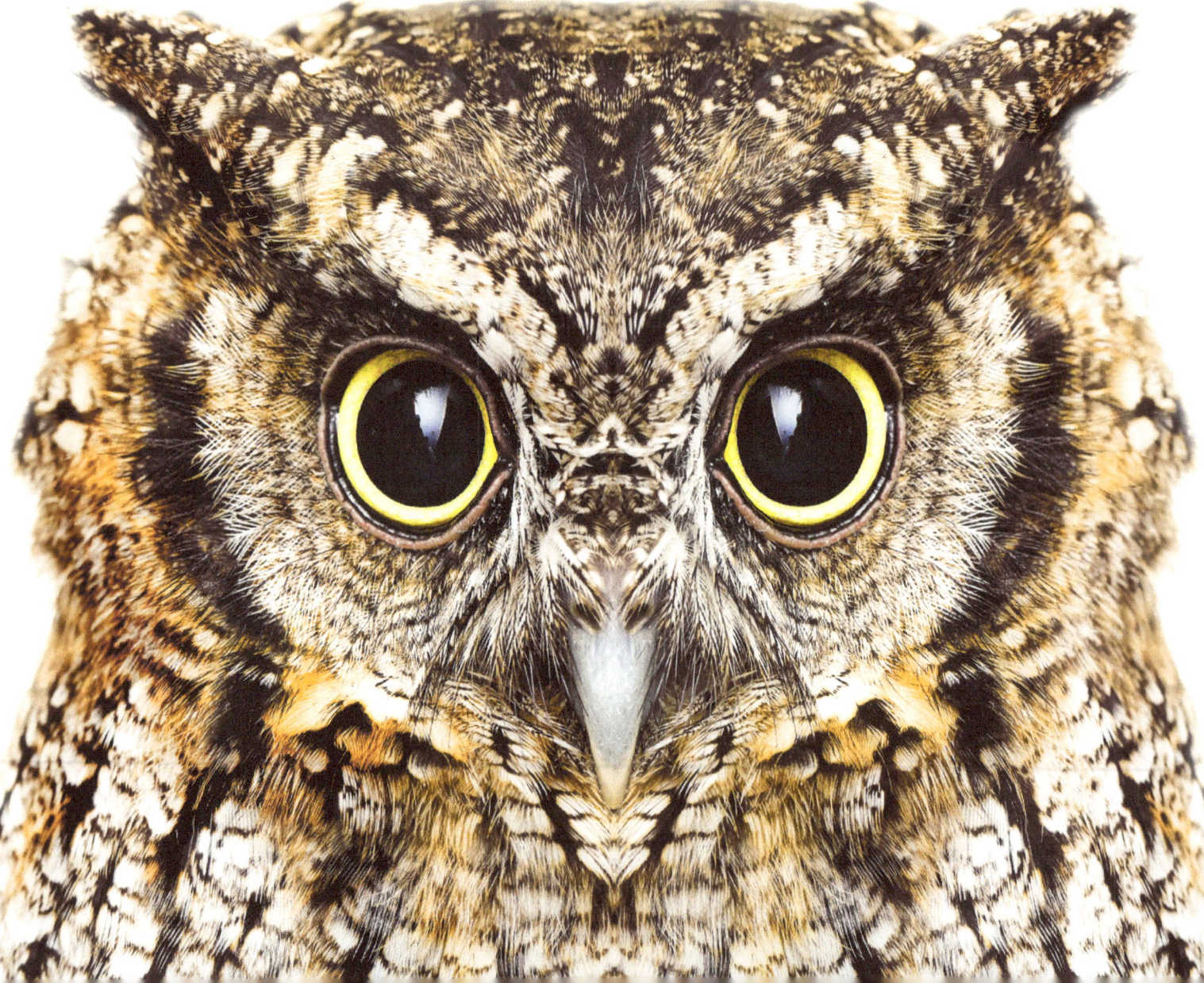

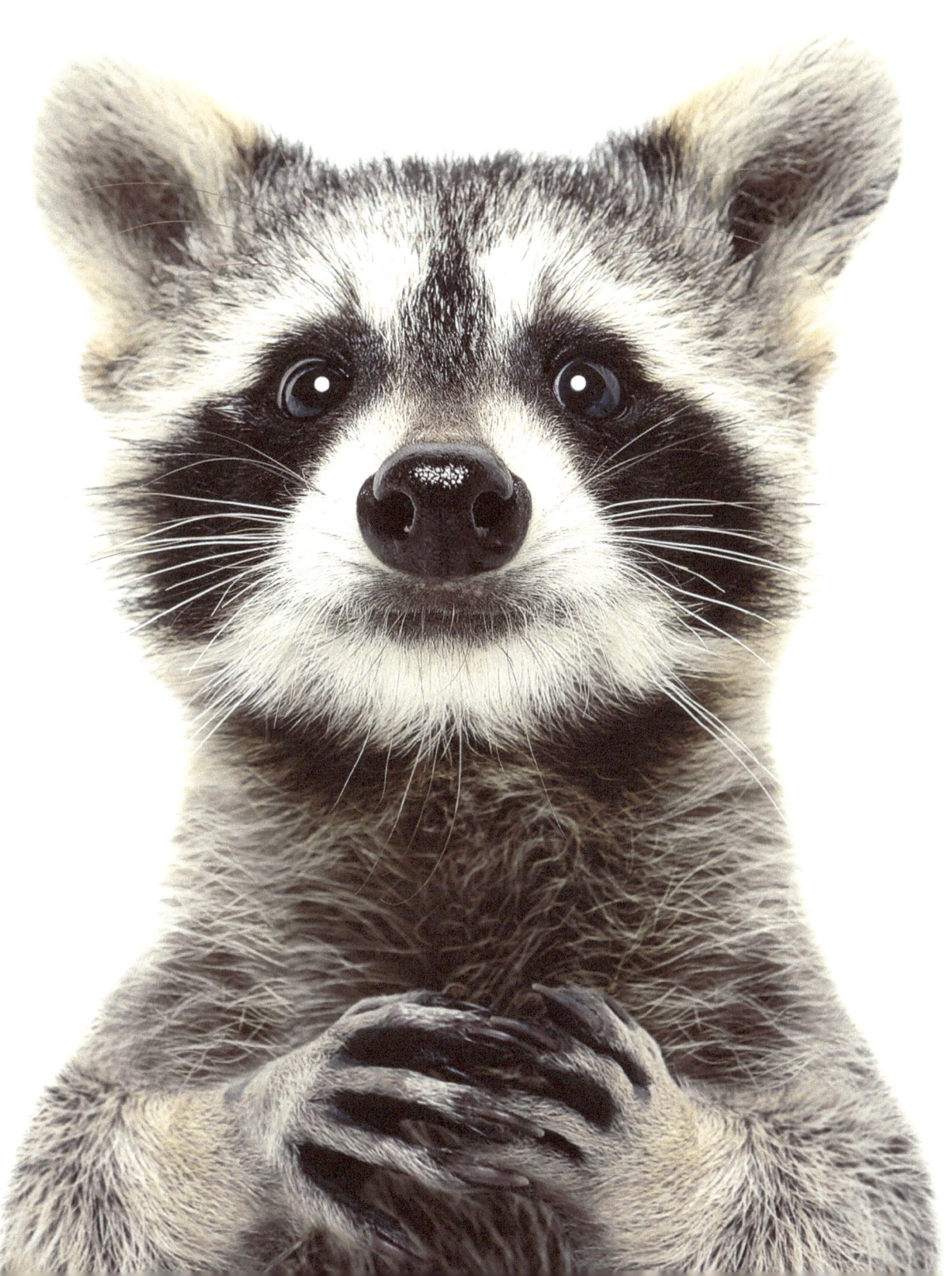

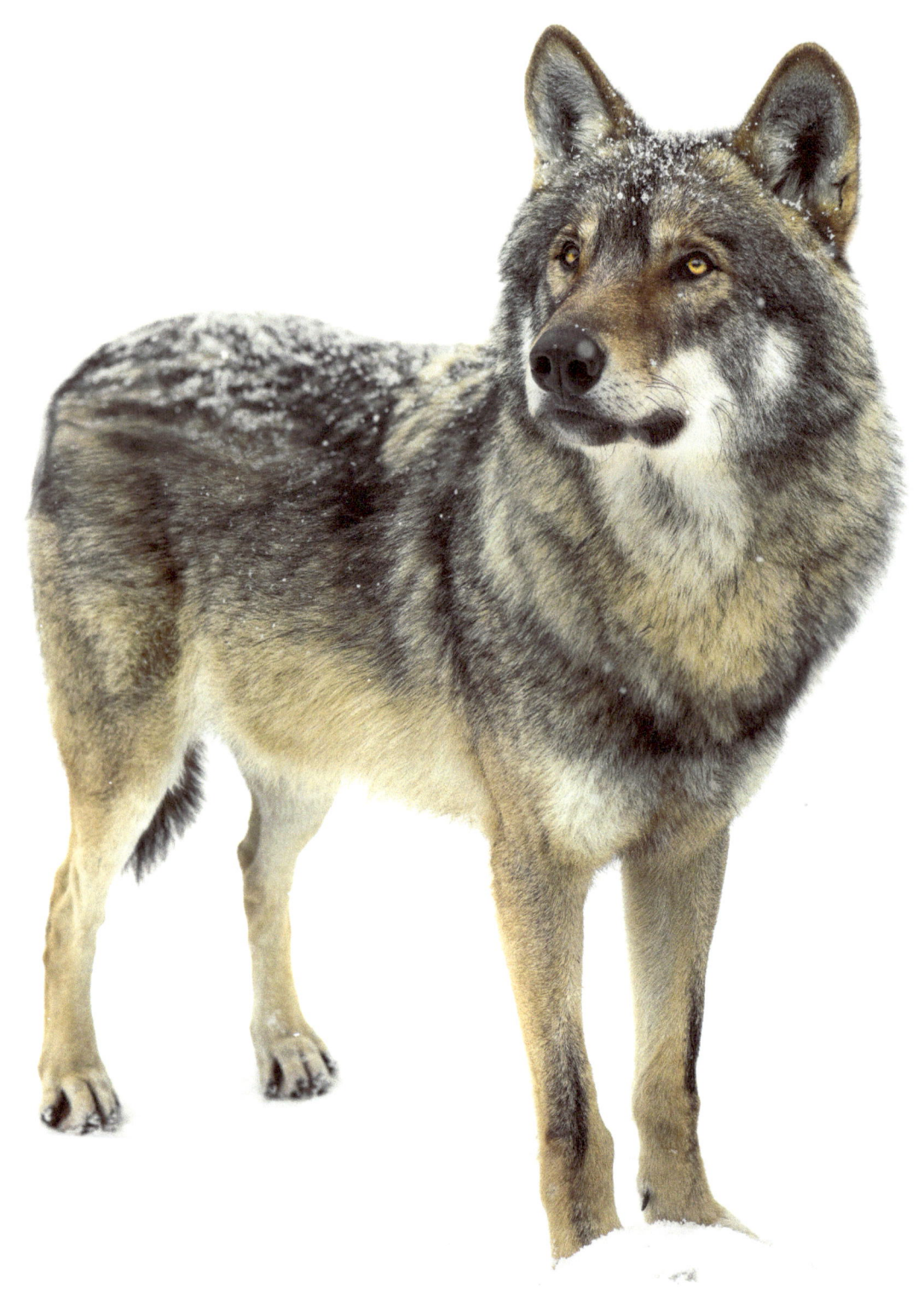

Lightning Source UK Ltd.
Milton Keynes UK
UKHW020631011222
413022UK00003B/196